Clinical Research in Psychiatry: a Practical Guide

Clinical Research in Psychiatry: a Practical Guide

Stephen Curran
BSc MBchB MMedSc MRCPsych PhD
Consultant in Old Age Psychiatry, Fieldhead Hospital, Wakefield

and

Christopher J. Williams
BSc MBChB MMedSc MRCPsych
Senior Lecturer in Psychiatry; Honorary Consultant Psychiatrist,
St James's Hospital, Leeds

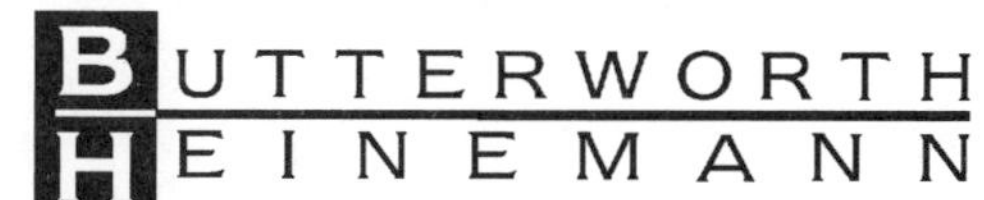

OXFORD AUCKLAND BOSTON JOHANNESBURG MELBOURNE NEW DELHI

Butterworth-Heinemann
Linacre House, Jordan Hill, Oxford OX2 8DP
225 Wildwood Avenue, Woburn, MA 01801-2041
A division of Reed Educational and Professional Publishing Ltd

A member of the Reed Elsevier plc group

First published 1999

British Library Cataloguing in Publication Data
A catalogue record for this book is available from the British Library

Library of Congress Cataloguing in Publication Data
A catalogue record for this book is available from the Library of Congress

ISBN 0 7506 4073 1

Typeset by Tek-Art, Croydon, Surrey
Printed and bound in Great Britain by Biddles Ltd,
Guildford and King's Lynn

Contents

List of contributors — *ix*

Foreword — *xi*

1 Why do research? — **1**
Philip Snaith
Introduction — 1
The place and function of research: the lessons of history — 1
The research cycle — 3
Making research interesting — 4
Beginning to undertake the research process — 5

2 Overcoming blocks to starting research — **9**
Christopher J. Williams
Introduction — 9
Why people do research — 10
Identifying blocks to starting research — 12
Overcoming your blocks to starting research — 15
Starting to do research: practical suggestions — 22

3 An introduction to research — **26**
David Richards and David West
Introduction — 26
The research question — 26
Stakeholders — 28
The project team — 29
Past and current research knowledge — 30
Choosing a methodology — 31
Reviewing the quality of the project — 35
Resources and costs — 37
Ethical issues — 39
Project management — 42
Dissemination — 44

4 Carrying out the literature search — **50**
Julie Glanville
Introduction — 50
The purpose of a literature review — 50
Defining the research question and budget issues — 52
Identifying resources to answer the question — 53
Carrying out the search — 58

Search issues 64
Data analysis and synthesis 66
Documenting the search 67
Conclusions 67

5 Writing a research protocol **70**
Stephen Curran
Introduction 70
Getting started – identifying the research question 71
Writing the protocol 74
The detailed content of the protocol 75

6 Descriptive statistics **83**
Tom Hughes
Introduction 83
Descriptive and inferential statistics 83
The different kinds of data 84
Properties of different kinds of data 84
Distribution 85
The normal distribution 85
Measures of average or 'central tendency' 86
Measures of spread 86
Deviations from 'normal': skew, kurtosis, more than one mode 88
Are my data normal? 89
The normal distribution and the standard deviation 90

7 Basic parametric statistics **91**
Amanda J. Farrin
Introduction 91
General structure of a statistical test 92
Setting up hypotheses 94
One sample *t*-test 95
Two sample *t*-test 96
Paired *t*-test 98
Computer software 100
Conclusions 101
Appendix 102

8 Basic non-parametric statistics **105**
Amanda J. Farrin
Introduction 105
Wilcoxon signed rank sum test 107

Mann-Whitney U test	109
Wilcoxon signed rank test (for paired data)	111
Computer software	112
Planning studies	113
Conclusions	113
Appendix	114

9 Using computers to facilitate research **117**
Patrick Harkin

Introduction	117
What are computers?	117
Choosing a computer	118
Research tasks which can be assisted by the use of a computer	120
Types of personal computers (PCs)	126
Computer viruses and other malicious software	126
Data security	129
Protecting yourself	132
Glossary	134

10 Maintaining momentum **138**
Anne Worrall-Davies

Introduction	138
Why you lose momentum	138
Overcoming obstacles to research: internal factors	139
Overcoming obstacles to research: external factors	144

11 Get it published! **147**
David Yeomans

Introduction	147
Why do I want to publish research?	147
Where to start?	148
Who is my audience?	148
Where can I publish?	149
What is a journal style?	150
How do I structure references?	151
How do I prepare the work for submission?	152
How do I get my paper to the journal?	153
How do I cope with reviews?	154
The final product	155

12 Ethical issues in research **157**
Ann Prothero
Introduction 157
Why submit research to an Ethics Committee? 157
Types of research which need to be submitted to an LREC 159
Issues considered during the review process 161
Recruitment of subjects 162
Information for participants 162
Consent 163
Confidentiality 164
Epidemiological research using medical records 164
Compensation for injury to research subjects 165
Deception 167

13 Obtaining research grants **170**
Julie L. Curran
Introduction 170
Sources of funding 171
Targeting your application 173
Contacting grant awarding bodies 174
How a grant is processed 174
Web sites, postal addresses and telephone numbers 176

Index *177*

Contributors

Julie L. Curran BSc (Hons), PhD
Clinical Scientist, St James's Hospital, Leeds; Visiting Research Fellow, Malignant Hyperthermia Investigation Unit, Research School of Medicine, Leeds University, Leeds

Stephen Curran BSc(Hons), MBChB, MMedSc, PhD, MRCPsych
Consultant in Old Age Psychiatry, Fieldhead Hospital, Wakefield

Amanda J. Farrin BSc, MSc
Research Fellow, Department of Health Sciences and Clinical Evaluation, University of York, York

Julie Glanville BA, MSc, PGDipLib
Information Service Manager, NHS Centre for Reviews and Dissemination, University of York, York

Patrick J. R. Harkin MB, ChB, BSc (Hons)
Lecturer in Pathology, University of Leeds, Leeds

Tom Hughes MRCPsych
Consultant Psychiatrist, High Royds Hospital, Leeds

Ann Prothero BSc (Hons)
Administrator, Clinical Research Ethics Committee, St James's University Hospital, Leeds

David Richards PhD, BSc (Hons)
Director of Research and Development, Leeds Community and Mental Health Services Trust, Meanwood Park Hospital, Leeds

R. Philip Snaith MD(Lond.), FRCPsych
Senior Lecturer in Psychiatry (retired), University of Leeds; Honorary Consultant Psychiatrist, St James's University Hospital, Leeds

David West BSc (Hons)
Research Tutor, Leeds Addiction Unit, Leeds

Christopher J. Williams MBChB, BSc (Hons), MMedSc, MRCPsych
Senior Lecturer in Psychiatry: Honorary Consultant Psychiatrist, St James's Hospital, Leeds

Anne Worrall-Davies MMedSc, MRCPsych, MD
Senior Lecturer in Child and Adolescent Psychiatry, University of Leeds, Leeds

David Yeomans BSc, MBChB, MMedSc, MRCPsych
Consultant Psychiatrist, Overthorpe House, Leeds

Foreword

Asking questions is one of the more enjoyable activities that we, humans, undertake. As psychiatrists we are fortunate to be employed to spend a large part of our working life asking questions. We refer to this as taking a psychiatric history, and it can be done well, with precision and following a comprehensive and orderly scheme, or badly.

There are also other question we need to ask. What is distinctive about this group of people we have been asked, as psychiatrists, to see? Are there any differences from others in their background? Does this treatment that we are using really work? If so, which components are essential for effectiveness? It is by this process of asking ever more refined questions that medicine, and psychiatry within it, has advanced. But there is considerable skill needed in asking such questions – and this is what this book is about. Research in psychiatry is the discipline of so asking and structuring our questions that we get answers that dependably contribute to the benefit of our patients.

The reader will find this to be a painless introduction to the essential building blocks of psychiatric research. It is consistently practical in nature, and addressed to the busy, clinically active, mental health practitioner. It offers thoughtful and professional advice on the major topics that will be encountered when starting research: carrying out a thorough and meaningful search of the literature, preparing a research protocol for funding, a substantial section on statistics applied to psychiatric research and the use of computers, the ethics of research, and how to obtain research grants.

It starts by posing the question that some psychiatric trainees have asked for decades – Why do research? – and goes on to discuss some of the reasons why mental health practitioners feel unable to get involved in research, and how to overcome this. A chapter on introduction to research runs, in a practical manner, through the various issues that a researcher will need to consider before embarking; many of these topics are dealt with more fully elsewhere in the book.

Appropriately, about three quarters of the way through the book comes a helpful chapter on maintaining momentum: why problems happen, and what to do about it when you run out of steam. The authors do not leave the reader with the finished product in limbo; there is a further practical chapter on getting the work published.

This is not a book for those who have already won a Nobel Prize for Medicine. The mental health researcher fully satisfied with the quality of their research and research output will find little of use. However, this is written for the rest of us who are still struggling to produce, to improve and to make our work relevant. It is commended to those in training in the mental health professions and also to those who take their own continuing professional development, as trained practitioners, seriously.

Andrew Sims

Chapter One

Why do research?

Philip Snaith

INTRODUCTION

The word 'research' will sound an alarming, even threatening note to many doctors commencing a medical career, especially a career in psychiatry – a branch of medicine often lacking in established benchmarks and where even the definitions of disorders are variable and constantly changing. There is therefore the temptation robustly to hang on to the opinions which appear to represent the view of 'established opinion'; to turn away from the vast chaos of opinion and uncertainty, to reflect perhaps with Omar Khayyám:

Myself, when young did eagerly frequent
Doctor and saint and heard great argument
About it and about: but evermore
Came out by the same door wherein I went.

But such a negative view of a questioning attitude serves neither science nor the art of psychiatric practice. Answers can be found concerning the nature and practice of psychiatry. The habit of questioning received opinion, or at least the opinion of one's teachers and seniors is sometimes discouraged or seen in a negative light as little more than presumption which is likely to irritate and hinder rather than help advancement – at least in respect to career progression.

THE PLACE AND FUNCTION OF RESEARCH: THE LESSONS OF HISTORY

The temptation is always to fit our clinical observations into the currently favoured theories of mental mechanisms, be these psychoanalytical or the reflexes of Pavlovian theory; or to retreat from all abstract theorizing of mental mechanisms and their disorders and rest one's faith on purely organic answers such as neuroanatomy, seeing altered brain function as the answer to all psychiatry's questions. There have been many occasions and examples in the history of psychiatry when claims have been made that there is no such concept as abnormal mental mechanism or 'disease of the mind' and to jettison these in favour of the view that mental illness is an invention to keep psychiatrists in employ and a means of individual and social oppression. Lest such a view be considered to be a recent phenomenon then read back more than a century to the heyday of institutional care; institutions then unashamedly termed lunatic asylums, and the efforts made in them to discover something of the nature and relief of their patients (Figure 1.1).

Figure 1.1 *Current thoughts on the practice of psychiatry*

'In the harmless, but vindictive, attacks which have been recently directed against the public lunatic asylums of this country, it has been a frequent charge that no scientific work is conducted in them. It has been an often repeated accusation that the medical officers of these establishments are so absorbed in general or fiscal management, in forming or in devising ill-judged amusements for their charges that they have no time or energy left to devote to professional research. And it has been further asserted that when these medical officers have by any chance ventured to enter the field of original investigation, they have, as a rule, signally failed to achieve any useful result because they are blinded and misled by erroneous method and by philosophical phantasms which their censors are of course presumed to possess in pre-eminent degrees.

While no sympathy, or even toleration is felt for such unwarrantable statements, or for that incapacity or disappointment of which they are the offspring; for that ignorance which knows nothing of medical literature; for that shallow-mindedness which recognises in the beneficent government of a community only the degradation of the huckster; for that pusillanimity which evades all metaphysical considerations or for that pauperised scientific spirit which ignores everything save weights and measurements, still a belief is entertained that there has perhaps been some remissness on the part of those engaged in the superintendance of our hospitals for the insane in publishing the results of their observations and contributing in proportion to their opportunities, their full share to our stock of precise knowledge . . .

That there has been any slackness on the part of asylum medical officers in completing the full role of professional duty in accordance with this high standard, has been to a certain extent due, not merely to the engrossing and exhausting character of these occupations which have properly filled the first place in their attention, but also to the absence of any immediate stimulus to this arrangement and elaboration of materials collected, and to want of any ready channel of exposition.

It is with view to supplying this deficiency and of affording the utilisation of much valuable information hitherto buried in case-books and diaries, that the present volume has been projected.'

The 'present volume' indicated in this quotation is in fact the series of *The West Riding Lunatic Asylum Medical Reports* which the writer, J. Crichton Browne initiated, edited and encouraged all members of the medical staff to contribute to.

It is important to consider how medical practice has changed over the last century and to ponder on the factors that have allowed such change. A good illustration of this can be found in the intermittent articles in the *British Medical Journal* which re-print in part or whole articles or comments about practice one hundred years ago. We might also consider how psychiatry will change over the next one hundred years. How much of our current practice will then seem ridiculously antiquated and missing the point? The purpose of these questions is to raise a number of very important issues:

- Why do we carry out our clinical practice as we do?
- Do current classification and treatment approaches make sense and explain the clinical presentations of the patients that we see every day, and if they do, do they actually help people get better?
- What are the most effective treatments for the disorders that we see? How do we decide which patients are likely to benefit the most from the treatments on offer?
- How do we learn and develop new practice? How do we change?

Underlying many of these questions is a far more important one – *how is progress made* in psychiatry or any other branch of medicine?

THE RESEARCH CYCLE

The nature of the scientific process involves a constant cycle of trying to make sense of our clinical practice. This *trying to make sense of things* involves attempts to formulate a theory or way of understanding the world or at least the part of the world that we work in – in the case of psychiatry, the patients we treat and have experience of. The research process involves a *cycle* of constant questioning of theory as it applies to practice. As we train as doctors and specialize in psychiatry, we read books and learn accepted theory. This leads to an understanding which allows specific hypotheses or predictions to be tested. The ability of our current models of understanding to reflect experience (e.g. to predict the outcome of different treatments) provides an indication of whether the theory is an adequate one. If they fail to explain findings, the implications are that they need to be altered (sometimes radically) and revisions proposed. This process of constant evolution is part of the process of clinical advancement and is illustrated in Figure 1.2. It is also very much the domain of everyday clinicians as well as full-time researchers.

Figure 1.2 *The research cycle: advancing clinical practice*

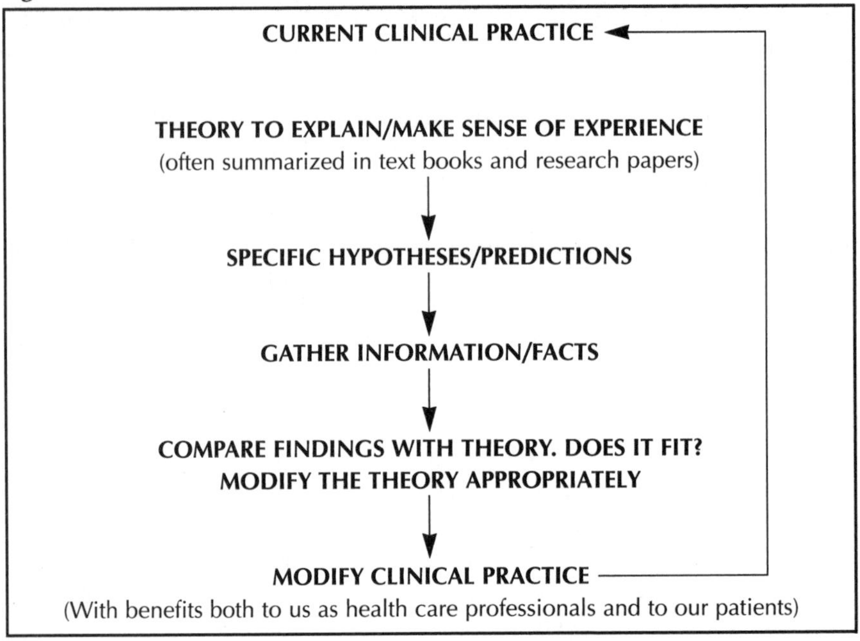

CURRENT CLINICAL PRACTICE ←

THEORY TO EXPLAIN/MAKE SENSE OF EXPERIENCE
(often summarized in text books and research papers)

↓

SPECIFIC HYPOTHESES/PREDICTIONS

↓

GATHER INFORMATION/FACTS

↓

COMPARE FINDINGS WITH THEORY. DOES IT FIT?
MODIFY THE THEORY APPROPRIATELY

↓

MODIFY CLINICAL PRACTICE →
(With benefits both to us as health care professionals and to our patients)

Those with an interest in the historical background of psychiatry might find that a visit to one or more of the medical museums that have developed at various hospital sites to retain records, equipment and the paraphenalia of past practice might help you understand your present practice in a different perspective.

MAKING RESEARCH INTERESTING

An important reason for questioning current practice by carrying out research at an early stage is that it can increase *interest* and provide *variety* in addition to the routine of clinical work. For instance, the assessment of people who deliberately and repeatedly harm themselves may sometimes appear to be a routine and, at times, frustrating task. It can be made more interesting by considering questions such as *why do people take overdoses*? Is it possible they suffer from recurrent brief depressive disorder? What percentage have seen a mental health worker recently, and if not, why not? For example, the enquiry as to what proportion of these attenders at a casualty department fit the criteria for recurrent brief depressive disorder would lead, not to an avoidance of, but to the request to be informed of such incidents so that the prevalence and impact of this disorder could be identified. Another example would be the observation in the behavioural therapy of phobic disorders of what proportion of such patients improved with an initial relaxation training programme with and without the element of exposure to the feared situation.

BEGINNING TO UNDERTAKE THE RESEARCH PROCESS

The concept of 'research' may conjure up thoughts concerning obtaining funding, the need for research assistance, dedicated time, specialist facilities and so on; all these will inhibit the trainee clinician – whether at commencement of training in psychiatry or later. The best procedure to overcome such blocks is to adopt at an early stage:

- A simple project.
- A line of enquiry into some clinical or other point which may be conducted in the setting of routine work and which may be conducted alongside your current work.
- A project achievable using the resources available to you.
- Anticipation of the impact of changes of job every six months on your ability to complete your work if you choose to work with others. A project which depends upon group activity, although perhaps enthusiastically adopted by all at the commencement, may later fall apart unless this problem is anticipated and planned for.

Some interest in the project and support from a tutor or other senior member of staff is helpful and potential difficulties in conducting the enquiry may be pointed out. However, it should be clear that the project is one's own initiative. If the starting point is that of an interest in the research area by the senior member of staff, then their helpful contribution may be welcomed. *It is important to try to avoid doing research (particularly at an early stage) which is someone else's idea rather than your own* and for which you have little personal enthusiasm. This may well affect your experience of research in the initial project and might later affect your subsequent attitude to and practice of research throughout your later training and clinical life. These issues are dealt with in greater depth in Chapter 2.

A key to successful research is to select an area which is of personal interest to you. A first useful step might be to think about those aspects of the research process in which you are currently involved. If you are at the stage of wanting to find out more about research, it can be useful to attend and consider the activity and lines of enquiry carried out as part of audit work within the hospital or Trust. The major purpose of audit is to investigate clinical activity and frequently an aspect of such enquiry can benefit from closer observation or development. The process of developing a research question and making it practical is outlined in Chapter 3.

The various literature retrieval systems, MEDLINE, PsycLIT and others are essential in carrying out a survey of any potential research topic and, if not already familiar with their use, the trainee should seek to gain skills in using these. Staff in hospital libraries are usually helpful in demonstrating the procedure for searches of subject headings or text words. The carrying out of such searches will lead to a vast amount of information – much of it of only marginal interest – but there will be some relevant publications. Indeed, a research project may simply be to carry out a systematic critical review of the current literature on a topic that has attracted your attention. With few exceptions it is possible to 'go beyond the textbook' to create an up-to-date enquiry on any topic. The exercise of adding one's own comment to a summary of these views is perhaps the most important aid in the development of clearer thought which will lead to a subsequent more meaningful enquiry into the topic.

The process of carrying out a literature review is summarized in Chapter 4. Other practical aspects of carrying out and completing the research process including how to clarify your ideas on research, decide on a focused research question, formulate a clear research plan (or protocol) and carry out your research are described in Chapters 5–9. Maintaining momentum is a key part of successful research. It is important not to lose your motivation during longer research activity. A number of practical self-help strategies to aid you through the crisis of research which has become 'stuck' are summarized in Chapter 10.

One purpose, although not necessarily the only reason for thought and observation on a project, is eventually to communicate your conclusions to other clinicians. Trying to *publish* your findings and get it into the public domain is a central process in the research cycle. It is by disseminating your findings that changes in current practice occur. Attempts to achieve publication in a major journal will, however experienced the researcher, often meet with rejection and discouragement. This can often be overcome if your initial sights are set somewhat lower, by for instance seeking publication as a brief communication, a letter to the Editor of a relevant journal or an inclusion in the Newsheet of the local Health Authority or Trust. Even here, rejection does not indicate a waste of effort. Chapter 11 describes the process of seeking publication. Even if a paper is rejected, you may receive some useful feedback suggesting clear things which may improve the design or content of your research. You can always learn from these experiences and use this new knowledge to modify your current and future research. Most important however, is that a process of critical enquiry will have commenced. This enquiring attitude should not be abandoned for it will add to the interest of your professional activity.

Progress in genuine knowledge of psychiatric practice is slow but constantly developing. The impediments to progress in psychiatric knowledge include:[1]

- Dogma – a standpoint which admits to no alternative view.
- Terminology – a penchant for using words, supposedly of some clinical significance, in such a variety of ways that clear scientific communication is lost: such diverse use is applied to terms such as 'depression', 'psychopath' and 'hysteria'.
- A system of classification based upon lists of symptoms from which any selection is admissible in order to apply the category.
- Measurement: scientific communication depends ultimately upon exact measurement but too often the scales used for measurement in psychiatric research are composed of such a medley of items that a high score would be achieved in most forms of ill-health. For instance, in two papers,[2, 3] the variation of disorder 'measured' by scales, all purporting to indicate the severity of 'depression' and of 'anxiety', were compared and found to be widely different in their content and purpose.

These confusions in psychiatric research should however not deter the trainee from commencing enquiry but should encourage more critical thought about the topic.

Much of the best research comes from asking 'why', 'how', 'when'. Much of the best research stems from clinical observations and questions. Many of the best researchers are also good clinicians. Clinical practice can only change by asking these and other questions. It is important to question current practices and beliefs. As you go through your clinical training, ask 'Is current theory accurate in my own experience?' If it isn't, you have the opportunity to ask your own questions and modify current theory and practice. Because of this, even small research studies can be very important. If you have such a research question, do something about it. You will find it challenging and potentially very rewarding. This book will help to show you how.

KEY POINTS

- You need to do research which *you* find personally interesting. Even small research studies can be interesting and important.
- Current clinical practice has evolved as part of a *research cycle* which involves constantly evaluating and re-evaluating our understanding of current clinical practice. You can contribute to this cycle.
- Begin by developing a project that can be done alongside your everyday work.
- Avoid doing research which is someone else's idea rather than your own.
- Publish your results. It is by disseminating your findings that changes in current practice occur.

REFERENCES

1. Snaith, R. P. Psychiatry is more than a science (corresp). *British Journal of Psychiatry*, 1993; **162**, 843–44.
2. Snaith R. P. What do depression scales measure? *British Journal of Psychiatry*, 1993; **163**, 293–98.
3. Keedwell, P., Snaith R.P. What do anxiety scales measure? *Acta Psychiatrica Scandinavica*, 1996; **93**, 177–80.

Chapter Two

Overcoming blocks to starting research

Christopher J. Williams

INTRODUCTION

Trainees in psychiatry often find themselves in an invidious position when it comes to doing research. A potent range of pressures encourage them to carry out research, yet it can seem very difficult to know even where to start the research process. This chapter is predominantly aimed at trainee psychiatrists who are starting out in the research process for the first time. It will help you identify your own blocks to research, and begin to plan out ways of overcoming them.

Positive pressures to do research come from different sources including:

- The Royal College of Psychiatrists: the Royal College requires all senior trainees to take part in research as part of their Higher training.[1] All UK specialist registrar (SpR) rotations in psychiatry put aside one day (two sessions) a week as 'protected' time for use in either research or further study. This is in addition to the time allocated for the clinical 'special interest' session.
- The local rotational training sub-committee: local SpR training schemes are regularly assessed by the Royal College to ensure that an appropriate range of training experience is available to trainees. This must include a balance of clinical work, management experience and research training or activity. Increasingly, opportunities for trainee research are being assessed by Royal College assessors and by postgraduate deans, training scheme organizers and others who wish to ensure that trainees can justify their use of the research/study day.
- University course organizers, (such as MMedSc or MPhil degrees). Many rotational training schemes now offer (often compulsory) attendance on a local postgraduate training course in psychiatry. These courses often include a mandatory research component.

Whereas the more academically inclined tend to find it easy to engage in research activity, for most, however, research will be done only sporadically and reluctantly. Few will publish more than one letter or short article even at the end of their specialist training. It is important to try to understand:

- Your motivation to do research.
- What pitfalls prevent research being started.
- What problems prevent research being completed.

In order to examine this, a recent survey of all senior trainees in the Northern and Yorkshire Region examined what research SpRs in psychiatry do.[2] This used a postal survey to investigate how senior trainees use their allocated research time, and to identify specific difficulties that prevent successful research being carried out. A standardized questionnaire was sent out in August, 1995 to all senior registrars working within all specialities of psychiatry within the Yorkshire and Northern Region. The questionnaire could be completed anonymously and was made up of five sections:

1. General demographic information: current and previous jobs and whether they were full or part-time.
2. Current research activity: including an assessment of the different factors that motivate people to do research, the time span of any research project, whether this was registered with a university, and assessed how many research sessions were taken each month over the last year.
3. Practical difficulties with research: this examined what practical problems have hindered research (e.g. lack of time, uncertainty how to proceed, lack of active support and lack of own interest).
4. Access to research resources: computer, word processor, statistical advice etc. and ability and confidence in using these.
5. Supervision and training: access to supervision and formal research training.

A total of 99 questionnaires were sent out and 57 (58%) questionnaires were returned; 79% of the responses were from full time senior registrars, and 21% part time. The study identified many of the issues that concern doctors when they start to do research and these are discussed in detail later in this chapter. It also examined the different motivations involved in influencing why trainees do research.

WHY PEOPLE DO RESEARCH

For trainees in many non-psychiatric specialities, research is necessary in order to advance through the training grades and attain an acceptable final job. For example, it is normal for trainee surgeons and physicians to complete a postgraduate research degree before they can obtain a consultant post. This is not the case in psychiatry. A quick look through the *British Medical Journal* classified advertisements each week will confirm the demand for psychiatrists in the UK and abroad. Many trainees will have friends or colleagues who obtain jobs at SpR or consultant level after publishing few if any articles. Why then do research? What is the point?

The study found that 48 (84.2%) of trainees in the Northern and Yorkshire Region were actively involved in some form of research, and only nine (15.8%) stated that they were doing no research. They pointed to a range of motivations for carrying out research and these are summarized in Table 2.1.

Table 2.1 *Motivation to do research*

Own interest	19 (33.3%)
CV purposes	17 (29.8%)
Advance career	13 (22.8%)
To please others	1 (1.8%)
Missing data	1 (1.8%)

It is clear from these findings that personal interest and pragmatic issues to do with enhancing career prospects are the two strongest motivating factors leading to research. Research *can* be very interesting, rewarding and creative. Evidence suggests that publications on CV are associated with success at job interview. [3,4]

Other factors can also make research attractive to junior doctors.[5] Research will enable you to:

- Learn new skills including specific skills in research methodology, research design and data analysis.
- Develop a specialized knowledge of a focused area in psychiatry. This may be useful clinically. In addition, you will gain in your understanding and practice of statistics and research design.

Research activity can also lead to additional non-research related benefits. A range of important generalizable skills can be developed. You will:

- Be able to think clearly and seek answers to specific questions.
- Develop a questioning attitude so that you can begin to avoid accepting statements at face value but instead begin to question evidence and current practice. You will begin to be able to evaluate research critically and determine its relevance to clinical practice. This has direct benefits for the new critical appraisal component of the Part II exam. It is likely that this will be increasingly important in the MRCPsych exams.
- Develop general writing and presentation skills (again useful for essays and exams).

- Enhance your ability to work independently and as part of a team. Working with others on collaborative research will help you develop management, organizational and leadership skills.
- Learn how to use library facilities/carry out a literature review and develop skills in the use of new technology/computer data analysis and word processing packages. Many doctors find that the process of carrying out research means that they have to use a computer for the first time. This can open up opportunities that will be useful both at home and work.
- Gain an insight into the practical application and difficulties in carrying out evidence-based approaches to clinical care. Actively doing research will alert you to opportunities for the development of a more evidence-based approach in your own clinical work setting.

From this brief review, it is clear that there are many potential benefits to research. Why then is it so rarely done well? Perhaps, sometimes, the positive aspects of research may be muddied by mixed motivations (such as doing the research for others rather than for oneself, the need for job references and the pragmatic desire to have a publication on one's CV). The survey identified a number of other blocks commonly encountered by those beginning to do research.

IDENTIFYING BLOCKS TO STARTING RESEARCH

The survey found that 60.7% of full-time trainees spent six or less sessions per month carrying out research with only 38.6% taking their full allocation of sessions. Only 21.1% reported a lack of interest as the main reason why their research was being hindered. Overall, 61.4% of trainees identified specific problems with carrying out research. The main problems identified are summarized in Table 2.2

Table 2.2 *Problems that have stopped or hindered research*

Lack of time	52.6%
Uncertainty how to proceed	47.4%
Lack of support from senior staff	29.8%
Lack of resources	29.8%
Own lack of interest	21.1%
Put off by the idea of writing a protocol	12.3%

1. Lack of time

There was widespread ignorance about the correct entitlement to research time. The majority (49; 86.0%) incorrectly stated that they were entitled to only one session of research a week. The correct entitlement is two sessions, allowing eight sessions of research a month for full-time SpR trainees. The allocation is half this for part-time trainees.[1] A majority (54.4%) found that clinical commitments restricted the amount of time they could allocate to planning or doing research. Reasons for this included:

- Difficulties balancing competing clinical and other demands: busy jobs with other pressures (e.g. to pass exams) can cause research to be squeezed out.
- A lack of formalized 'protected' time specifically put aside for research: this problem was particularly acute for part-time trainees.
- Inappropriate expectations by consultants: sometimes individual consultants expect supernumerary SpRs to attend ward rounds, clinic sessions or provide cover at all times when the consultant is away. Some unfortunately seem actively to discourage research or seem neutral about it. Some may attempt to 'use' your research time and enthusiasm to do time-consuming and unrewarding work. This is clearly inappropriate. SpRs are doing their job when they take their research sessions. The trainer risks losing their training status if they actively discourage research or act to prevent you taking these sessions. Most are aware of this, and tactful approaches to the trainer to discuss the balance or content of the job, or direct contact with the scheme organizer is likely to rectify the situation. It is rarely necessary for the Royal College to be directly involved.

2. Uncertainty how to proceed and lack of access to resources

Uncertainty how to proceed with research is common. Unfortunately, many MMedSc and MPhil courses do not adequately prepare trainees to carry out their own research. Problems can include:

- Having no ideas for research of your own.
- A lack of skills in research methodology and therefore not knowing how to start.
- A lack of access to local doctors with research experience who can help plan and facilitate your research.
- A lack of secretarial support or a lack of even the minimal financial support needed to proceed with a project can be a major block to research.
- A lack of other important research resources such as access to computers, word processing and statistical software can also be important. It is not enough to have access to computers alone. In the survey, although 46 (80.7%) had access to a computer, between 66.7% and 84.2% felt that they did not have the skills necessary to use a computer, word processor or carry out a CD-ROM literature review;

64.9% could not use a statistical package. Actively doing some research can therefore be an opportunity for learning these skills. This is often the first time that doctors have had to use a computer. This problem can be overcome if the right support is available, however, it can be off-putting if there seems to be little support.

3. Lack of interest and ambivalence towards research

Ambivalent feelings often arise when trainee psychiatrists begin to think about becoming involved in research. External pressures such as the views of the Royal College, rotational scheme organizers and others may seem unimportant compared with the need to pass Part I or II College exams. Exams and other aspects of life outside work are important. Ask yourself:

- Who is the research for? Motivation will be less if it is perceived that the work is being done for someone else rather than because it is of interest to you. This is often a cardinal mistake.
- Is the time right? When you choose to carry out research is important. Seek the right balance when it comes to deciding when to carry out research. Different types of research are appropriate at different times in your career. This is discussed in greater detail later in this chapter.

4. Peer group pressures and the anti-research social milieu

The influence of others in a rotational scheme or in a hospital setting can have a marked impact. Even among insightful psychiatrists, the social pressures to conform can be potent. Peer pressure affects our patients, it also affects us. There can be a powerful 'canteen' culture in certain hospitals which labels research as 'hard' or 'boring'. This can be a potent force against becoming involved. When was the last time you had a conversation with someone over lunch about a good research idea you have had? Would the idea of this make you feel uncomfortable? What would others say? If you fear that this would adversely affect how others see you, then perhaps peer pressures are affecting your own attitude to research.

5. Does research seem irrelevant?

Many have found that their medical school training has left them ill prepared to think or question their clinical practice. Unfortunately, the way that medicine is often taught teaches us the lesson that the way to success is most easily found through rote learning of information delivered in lectures or books. This must be learned so that the hurdle of the next exam can be leaped. The result is that trainee doctors may see research as something that is irrelevant or as something that might act to block your career progression rather than something they can actively be involved in and direct themselves.

6. A fear of the implications of research

Sometimes people's perception of research can almost amount to a 'research phobia'. Research becomes the 'R' word that cannot be spoken.[5] Trainees often may have ambivalent feelings about research. In order to identify your own thoughts about research, spend a minute or so now jotting down whatever thoughts come into your own mind when you think about the idea of carrying out research.

- What are my chances of succeeding if I start to do research?
- How easy will it be for me to decide on a clear research question?
- Will I be able to work through the research process?
- Would I be able to approach analysing the data?
- Do I have a clear idea how I will write up and publish the results?

7. The impact of life changes

Your individual social situation can also affect your motivation to do research. Life events such as moving office, looking for new jobs every few months, developing a new relationship, decorating the house etc., can all make research seem like an added burden. This has implications for your job plan and the timing and extent of your research.

8. The effect of full time/part time employment on research

Time pressures are particularly acute for part-time trainees. Part-time trainees are entitled to one research session (half a day) a week. In the survey, part-time senior registrars experienced significantly more difficulties carrying out their research as a result of clinical work (chi squared – 3.88, 1 df; $P<0.05$). They took less time for research and found it more difficult protecting this time.

9. Procrastination: putting it off

Sometimes procrastination becomes a major issue when it comes to carrying out research. It is important for you to deal with this. Is the problem specific to this research problem or is it a problem that you have in many other areas of life? The next section of the chapter will look at ways of improving your motivation and of planning how to overcome your problems of procrastination in a step-by-step manner.

OVERCOMING YOUR BLOCKS TO STARTING RESEARCH

Complete the checklist in Table 2.3 to identify which of the seven areas you have problems addressing.

***Table 2.3** Assessing blocks to your research*

Checklist identifying blocks to starting to do research:		
1. Too little time/disrupted by job pressures	Yes	No
2. Uncertainty how to begin	Yes	No
3. Lack of research skills or lack of expert support	Yes	No
4. Lack of resources (computer, money, secretarial support)	Yes	No
5. Poor motivation/ambivalence	Yes	No
6. Negative view of research by you or peers	Yes	No
7. Procrastination – putting it off	Yes	No

How to overcome these blocks/difficulties

1. Too little time/disrupted by job pressures

- Choose the right time to do research: for the first year or so in psychiatric practice, trainees often tend to focus on learning skills of clinical assessment and diagnosis in order to pass the Part I MRCPsych exam.[6] Choosing the right time to start research is therefore important. Many find that the gap between Part I and II exams is a good time to start carrying out smaller research topics such as writing a case report etc. This allows other areas rather than just the learning of academic facts to be developed. This can include gaining new clinical skills as well as research skills. Completing some small, focused research projects at this time means that by the time Part II is passed, it is possible to develop further research skills that already exist. After successfully obtaining an SpR post, you will then have access to a dedicated day to further your research and build on your knowledge.
- Prioritize the work you want to do: it may be that you wish to take a long-term view. The SpR rotation normally lasts for 3 years. During this time, you need to gain clinical skills and management experience and do some research. If you can, think about having a long-term plan to allow you to cover each of these areas adequately.
- Build research into your job plan: make sure that when you enter each job there is an opportunity to discuss your research as well as your clinical needs. According to the Trainees charter,[7] at least one hour a week should be given over to discussion of your non-clinical needs. This provides an opportunity to discuss your research. It can also help you identify useful local supports and resources to help you with the research you wish to do.
- Part-time trainees: if you are a part-time trainee, there is a particular need for you to make sure that your research time is protected. Many find it is easier to set aside a whole day for research every fortnight rather than unsuccessfully attempting to protect half a day each week. Discuss this with your consultant and supervisor. They will realize the difficulties of working part-time and should be able to offer you positive

support in this. Try to make changes that allow you to protect your research sessions. If you are officially using one of your research sessions, try to ensure that the wards, secretary and your consultant know this and that you are not to be contacted. Switch your bleep off and inform others (including switchboard) so that there are no misunderstandings.

2. Uncertainty how to begin

Much of the best research stems from interesting clinical observations or questions. Good research skills, like good clinical skills require time, practice and supervision to develop. If you find that you have very few ideas of what to do with your research time, there are a number of potential first targets including small research projects that will help you build your research skills one step at a time. Look for research ideas in your everyday life. These can include:

- Case reports: what interesting or unusual patients have you come across on the wards? For example, Dr Barry Wright has written up the case of a man who presented to casualty with mania after sleep depriving himself for four days. Sleep-deprivation had been previously described as a cause of mania, and there is a small literature on this. The rarity made the case publishable and it was published within the *British Journal of Psychiatry*.[8]
- Consider writing a review: summarizing current information about a topic will help you with your exams and also provide an area of knowledge which may be developed into further research or potential publications in the field, thus achieving several benefits from the initial work. If you wish to do this, it is best to seek out a senior colleague with expertise in the field and to collaborate with him or her.
- Questions about clinical or ethical practice: from time to time all clinicians find that they face difficult dilemmas in their practice of psychiatry. For example, two patients came into casualty, both of whom suffered from psychiatric disorders which left them unable to either consent or withhold consent from treatment. Both needed surgical operations to save their lives. This is an important clinical issue which tends to present to non-psychiatrists. This case was published in the *Journal of the Royal Society of Medicine*.[9]
- Surveys of knowledge/attitudes or current clinical delivery: for example, the survey of SpRs' attitudes and practice of research described in this chapter and numerous other surveys published for example in *Psychiatric Bulletin*.
- An area of interest: if you are interested for example in electroconvulsive therapy and keep abreast with the key past and current literature, you will find that you are quickly able to write letters commenting on current newsworthy events in this area, review the research work of others, write about recent advances or current trends

and develop your own research reputation in this area. You could then go on to produce updated publications in the same field every few years and become a recognized expert.

- A reaction to something else: if you read someone else's article or research, sometimes this can spark off an interest and cause you to want to investigate further. Sometimes an interesting research article, conference presentation or journal club discussion may stimulate your own interest. If you have such a research idea, write it down to prevent you forgetting it. Talking it through with others will help you to focus on the research question and make sure that it is clear, focused and attainable (see Chapter 3).

3. *A lack of research skills or expert support*

- Seek out research training: only 7% of trainees in the survey described their research training as 'good', with 52.6% describing their training as 'adequate'. Worryingly, 38.6% believed their training was 'poor' or 'non-existent'. A majority (63.2%) had received formal training in research methodology, and this had mostly been within the setting of local university courses (38.6%). Only 7% had attended a Royal College of Psychiatrists training course or workshop in research methodology. If you know that you lack a basic training in research or lack confidence in the process of starting to do research, plan to:
    - Read a good book on research (e.g. *Research methods in psychiatry: A beginners guide*[10]).
    - Go on a training day (local or national). The Royal College advertises one and two day research courses several times a year. Watch out for them in *Psychiatric Bulletin*. If you do attend a course, aim to go to it with a mind to developing further an existing research idea. Plan to carry through this idea in the few weeks after attending the course so that you put into practice what you have learned. This will help reinforce the skills you have gained.

4. *Lack of resources (computer, money etc.)*

Think about the advice you would give to a patient if they were faced with a practical problem like this at work. You might suggest that they adopt a problem-solving approach to try to overcome this difficulty.[11] You could help them to:

- Identify and clearly define the problem as precisely as possible, (e.g. no money to pay for stamps/ envelopes for a survey of clinical practice).
- Brainstorm multiple possible solutions to the problem. The more solutions you generate, the better (include ridiculous ideas as well initially), (e.g. are there any local Trust seedcorn moneys, does your university have a small student fund to encourage research. Is a small grant is available from a charity? Would a larger grant funding body

support it? Could you pay for it yourself? What about the rotational scheme organizer – do they have access to funds or information concerning other possible sources of financial support? What about your Trust Research and Development Unit? How about using the Trust internal mail system and transit envelopes to cut costs? Would a drug representative donate some money? Could you rob a bank?

- Assess how effective and practical each suggestion is. Which solution is most likely to be effective/ethical/practical and achievable? The idea of robbing a bank seems untenable, but perhaps deciding to seek a small grant from your local university course fulfills the criteria of being more likely to be successful and not overly difficult to put into action.
- Choose one of the solutions.
- Plan out the steps needed to carry it out, e.g. contact the local university secretary and ask if there are any grants or financial supports. Confirm what types of work they support, by whom, how much for and for how long. Ask for an application form and find out what information needs to be sent to whom and by when.
- Do it! Complete and submit the application form and send it in.
- Evaluate the outcome. Did it work? If it did, well done. Get the money and spend it on the project. If not, try to work out why. Could you have made the case any more persuasively? Was there any useful feedback from peer reviewers which made suggestions that you could put into a further or revised application? etc.

With flexibility, this approach can be used with any practical problem. For example, it is likely that somewhere near where you work there will be access to computers and training. Management training courses often offer training in word-processing and use of the Internet. Your local library will often give access and training in literature searching using CD-Roms. Most university courses will provide you with a computer username and access to the Internet, literature search facilities, libraries and computers. Discuss any practical problems concerning a lack of access to research resources with your tutor. No training scheme wants to gain a reputation for providing an inadequate training experience. Money can often be found to purchase appropriate equipment for use by trainees within medical libraries etc. If access is difficult, discuss this with your trainer and training scheme organizer. The Royal College will often support trainees' requests for additional resources in this area if they are sparse. Be inventive. Look for answers and you will normally find them.

5. *Poor motivation/ambivalence*

If you are uncertain about the reasons why research is important, it is important to consider the reasons why you would want to do research. Think about the advantages and disadvantages of doing research. Try to identify internal and external factors for and against your doing research now. Try to take a long-term perspective. If you put off doing research now, will you regret it in a year, or two years or in five years? What will the impact be on you, your skills, and your chances of promotion? Perhaps you do not wish to move through the career ladder towards a consultant post – if so, could research still be interesting for you? It can help to write down the costs and benefits for you of choosing to do research (Figure 2.1).

Figure 2.1

Benefits of research (now, later, for me, for others)	**Costs of research** (now, later, for me, for others)
1	1
2	2
3	3
4	4
5	5

6. Negative view of research by yourself or others

If you or your peer group believes that research is only for very intelligent achievers or the boring and obsessional, then it is important to question whether this is true. Are there any good researchers you know who are not like this? Do you know any respected teachers or clinicians who also do research? Is the stereotype true in your own experience? Even if it is, does this mean that you cannot change it? Many scientific breakthroughs have occurred as a result of people taking a different view from that held by the majority. Do you see yourself as being more of a clinician than a researcher? If you find that you are not doing things that you really wish to do because of the views of others, it is important to try to question why this is. Part of your training in becoming a consultant involves being clear about what you want to do and why. It is important for your own development to resist peer pressures. If you find that this is a major issue for you, considering reading a book on assertiveness or attending (or jointly running!) an assertiveness course. This may also help you in other areas of your life and be useful clinically when it comes to helping patients learn to change themselves.

What does research mean to you? The concept of research can mean many different things to different people. If research is defined narrowly as some high powered biological investigation or the 'gold-standard' placebo-controlled double-blind trial, then this often is beyond the reach of most trainees in their initial steps in doing research. These styles of research are probably best left to more senior researchers or clinicians who have a clear research focus which they pursue over some years. What 'research' then should trainees undertake? In Leeds, junior staff at pre-SpR level are first encouraged to become involved in small scale research projects such as surveys, writing a case report, or carrying out an audit before embarking on a larger scale research dissertation. These often flow from ideas they have when doing their clinical jobs. This work can be supervised and encouraged by a more senior and experienced colleague. The interest and enthusiasm must come primarily from the trainee. This can act as the first step in helping trainees think and work critically in their clinical practice.

7. Overcoming procrastination

If you find that you constantly put off starting research, this part of the chapter is for you. First, spend a little time sitting down and writing down what thoughts come into your mind when you think about starting to do research.

- Am I just too busy?
- Am I avoiding starting or even thinking about research?
- Do I see research as something that is just too large a thing to do?
- What does this say about how I see research?
- What does this say about me?

In order to overcome procrastination it is important to look at two main issues:

- Increasing my motivation. This was dealt with in point number 5.
- Planning to make changes one step at a time. A number of practical changes can be helpful in making your research more achievable.

Think about the right size of project. Start small. 'Research' can range from focused longer-term 'gold-standard' research projects through to smaller projects such as carrying out and writing up material at the level of case reports or small surveys which are achievable within 6–12 months, requiring minimal resources. This may be a first step in helping you think and work critically by including research in your clinical practice. If you feel overfaced by the idea of carrying out a large research project, it can sometimes be more helpful to think of research as a smaller 'clinical project'. These can include the case reports, surveys, letters and clinical audits described earlier in the chapter. Build up your confidence and skills with these first. They can sometimes act as a pilot project for a larger research project and may lay the foundation for a larger research project such as that which may be submitted for a higher degree such as an MD, MPhil, MMed Sc., or PhD.

STARTING TO DO RESEARCH: PRACTICAL SUGGESTIONS

What research do you want to do? If you are about to start out doing research, try to make it:

- Interesting.
- Relevant.
- Practical.
- Achievable.

What are achievable goals?

Early on in the research process, you need to decide whether to do research on a small scale or be prepared for the 'long haul' of a larger project. Whichever way you choose, for most trainees you will have to face the challenge of how to do research with:

- Little money.
- In your own time.
- In your normal job.

Before you start

Predict in advance what problems or difficulties may make planning or starting the research difficult.

- Think.
- Share: talk to as many people as possible.
- Set targets.
- Review progress: consider how you plan to start developing the research. What problems might occur. Look constructively at how to overcome any practical problems that might hold you back.
- Work with others: collaborative working offers many benefits and can help ensure that the work happens.

  This offers the advantages of:

- Mutual encouragement.
- Set deadlines of when tasks must be done or progress summaries given in order to focus your mind.
- Work with others with complementing skills (e.g. one person may be good at coming up with ideas, another at writing and another at statistics). Work to your strengths.

- Split the work up fairly. A larger research project can result from different component parts.
- One piece of research can therefore lead to a publication for a number of different people who all collaborated on the project.
- The presence of supportive supervisors or consultants can be a great help. It is likely that certain consultants will have a good local or national reputation in research. Seek them out and ask their advice. A further variant is for the trainee to try to link with an NHS consultant and academic psychiatrist in order to develop research projects and skills – the so-called research troika model.[12]

One practical way of creating an environment where each of these principles can helpfully aid research is to consider meeting with other like-minded doctors. One way of doing this is to form an informal research club.

Research clubs

'Juniors-only' research clubs can be a helpful way of working with others in a way that encourages research. The research club at St James's Hospital in Leeds meets once a month and lasts for 90 minutes.[5] Only staff at SpR level or below are allowed to attend, and this aims to defuse feelings of tension or stress that might otherwise be felt. A cycle of meetings is held every six months. This includes an introductory meeting that outlines the fact that research can be interesting, relevant and achievable in the limited time available to trainees. Presentations are made by peers who are currently carrying out small projects, and small group work is then used to brainstorm potential interesting research ideas and how to take them forward.

The junior doctors who come can choose to work individually or as part of a small group. By the end of the second meeting, each small group is encouraged to go away to gather more information and to write a protocol. These are then presented to the group for constructive criticism at the next club meeting. This approach can lead to the person wanting to take the questions they have asked further, perhaps in the form of a larger research project as part of a postgraduate research degree. This is an interesting and helpful way of integrating academic, clinical and research skills in a way which complement each other.

What can the College do?

Freeman (1992) has advocated the setting up of a network of College Research Training Coordinators to provide practical assistance and supervision for trainees engaging in research for the first time.

There is a need for consultants to seek out training in research design and supervision. The Research activity logbook suggested by the Joint Committee on Psychiatric Higher Training of the Royal College of

Psychiatrists will focus the minds of both trainees and trainers alike on the need for adequate research training and experience.

Finally, take heart from the publication in *Psychiatric Bulletin* by Peter McColl:[13]

> Dear Sirs, As a (first rate) post-membership registrar in an intensely busy post I have little enough time to put together an SR application let alone 'publish' for it. Hence this letter. Many thanks.

KEY POINTS

Make it interesting!

- Keep it small.
- Look for opportunities.
- Must be achievable/simple.
- Don't go over the top.

Do it with a friend!

- Complement each other's skills.
- Reduce the workload.
- Set achievable tasks and encourage progress together.

Beginning research:

- Think!
- Have clear targets which are achievable.
- Be motivated: make it happen.
- Talk and seek help from others who know about the research process.
- Consider setting up an informal research club so that you can encourage others and they can encourage you.

REFERENCES

1. Joint Committee on Higher Psychiatric Training Committee. *Joint Committee on Higher Psychiatric Training Committee, Handbook, 7th edn*, Occasional Paper OP/27. 1995; Royal College of Psychiatrists: London.
2. Williams, C. J., Curran, S. Research by senior registrars in psychiatry. *Psychiatric Bulletin*, 1998; **22** (2), 102–4.

3. Lewis, S. The right stuff? A prospective controlled trial of trainees' research. *Psychiatric Bulletin*, 1991; **15**, 478–80.
4. Katona, C. L. E., Roberston, M. M. Who makes it in psychiatry: CV predictors of success in training grades. *Psychiatric Bulletin*, 1993; **127**, 27–9.
5. Williams C. J., Curran, S. Should Psychiatric Trainees do research? *Psychiatric Bulletin*, 1996; **20**, 162–4.
6. Ferran, J. Publish or perish? *Psychiatric Bulletin*, 1993; **17** (6), 374.
7. Royal College of Psychiatrists Collegiate Trainees' Committee. Trainees' Charter. *Psychiatric Bulletin*, 1994; **18**, 440–2.
8. Wright, J. B. D. Mania following sleep deprivation. *British Journal of Psychiatry*, 1993; **163**, 679–80.
9. Porter S., Williams, C. J. Psychiatric dilemmas: surgery and the Mental Health Act (1983). *Journal of the Royal Society of Medicine*, 1997; **90**, 327–30.
10. Freeman, C., Tyrer, P. eds *Research Methods in Psychiatry: A Beginner's Guide*. 2nd edn. 1992; Gaskell: London.
11. Williams, C. J. Cognitive behaviour therapy. In: *Pass the MRCPsych Essay*, (Williams, C. J., Trigwell, P. J. eds). 1996; W. B. Saunders, London.
12. Sims, A. C. P. Research Troikas: a plan for fostering psychiatric research in a region. *Psychiatric Bulletin*, 1992; **16**, 605–7.
13. McColl, P. SR Posts and publications. *Psychiatric Bulletin*, 1993; **17**, 505.

Chapter Three

An introduction to research

David Richards and David West

INTRODUCTION

The purpose of this chapter is to describe the basic principles and potential pitfalls involved in starting to do research. Many of the chapters in this textbook will describe aspects of the research process in detail. This chapter will provide the framework within which research takes place. It covers essential aspects of the process including:

- Developing the research question.
- Placing the question in context.
- Identifying resources.
- Using research outcome management to implement the research project.
- Dissemination of findings.
- Practice change and audit.

THE RESEARCH QUESTION

The first stage in any research project is developing the research question. The best advice to any researcher is to ask the small question of the large area. Keeping the subject of the research project within manageable limits is the key to success and formulating the research question is the first stage in this discipline.

Research questions are, therefore, very important statements which also guide researchers in the choice of research method. Choices of question style are determined by:

- The subject of study.
- The philosophical orientation of the researcher.
- The study design.

Generally, *qualitative* researchers and surveys use questions whereas *quantitative* or experimental research poses hypotheses. Creswell[1] provides several models for research questions. Qualitative research (described later):

- Poses '*grand tour*' questions which are about discovery.
- Does not posit a causal relationship.
- Uses words like 'describe, discover, explore, explain'.
- Does not propose a relationship between variables.
- Does not differentiate between independent and dependent variables.

Beneath the grand tour questions are specific 'sub-questions' which delve into the specific areas of discovery. Here questions might begin with 'what, how, which'. Qualitative research reflects the researchers' ideals of discovering relationships and developing theories from these relationships.

In contrast, the research hypotheses used in quantitative research are derived from a positivistic view of science and are:

- Often developed from theory.
- Have separate elements for independent and dependent variables.
- Suggest a relationship (or lack of relationship) between variables.
- Reflect the experimental 'cause and effect' approach to science.

Traditionally researchers have been encouraged to use the *null hypotheses* (H_0) to structure their enquiry. Here the hypothesis is structured in such a way as to predict no relationship between variables and the experiment is designed to prove that no such relationship actually exists. For example, a research hypothesis might state that, 'There is no relationship between . . . (dependent variable *a* – e.g. age) and (independent variable *b* – e.g. depression) . . .' Such an approach drives statistical assumptions of significance where the null hypothesis can only be disproved when the scale of difference between two or more conditions is much greater than that which may occur by chance. Only when the null hypothesis is so dramatically disconfirmed can researchers assert that differences between groups are real.

Whatever the approach, all research questions or hypotheses should be:

- Clear.
- Precise.
- In simple language.

There may be more than one question or hypothesis, but all should state which population is to be researched and the context within which the research should take place. The reader of a research protocol must be very clear as to the objectives of the research and, having read the methods section, will know how the research is going to answer the questions posed. A good rule of thumb is that individual research questions should be no longer than 20 words.

STAKEHOLDERS

Before embarking on a piece of research work it is necessary for researchers to consider some fundamentals.

- Who is affected by the research?
- Who should be steering the research?
- Who should be doing the research?
- Will there be academic supervision?
- Who is going to pay for it?
- What are the financial limitations?

Considering these points, it is possible to identify the stakeholders in the research other than the researchers themselves, for example:

- Service users who will be 'subjects' (or more properly research 'participants').
- Organizations responsible for providing existing or proposed services to research participants.
- Owners, managers and users of any infrastructure connected with the research.
- Those who contribute to any processes being researched.
- Those contributing their expertise to the research process itself.
- Research funders.

Funders

Increasingly, funding for research comes through specially commissioned programmes in which there will be a detailed research brief put out by the funding agency (see Chapter 13 for more detailed information). This must be consulted and considered prior to developing a research project. When developing protocols and bids for such commissioning briefs it is worth asking the following questions:

- What are the commissioner's main research objectives?
- Is the research likely to meet these objectives?
- Is it possible to convince the commissioners that the project is deliverable in the proposed time frame, with the available resources and by the proposed research team?

We recommend that in larger or funded research projects researchers should consider setting up a *project steering group* consisting of representation from all the major stakeholders. This not only provides welcome advice but can also assist in keeping the project on track.

Conflicts of interest may arise between the needs of different stakeholders. Most obvious, though by no means the only example, is the conflict between commercial interests in the medical industry and the views of other stakeholders. Such conflicts are not necessarily wrong in themselves, but not openly acknowledging them would be. Careful consideration of real and potential conflicts of interest may help to ensure that the integrity of all concerned is maintained and that anyone reading the research report will not be inappropriately cynical of a commercially funded study.

THE PROJECT TEAM

There are two aspects to the team's constituency:

- The training and expertise of researchers and supervisors.
- Involvement of different professional groups (multi-disciplinary mix).

It is important that researchers are adequately trained for the research task.

- Funding bodies will require evidence that the team is competent and that there is at least some track record of research. Often, although a research team may be new to an area, it will be able to demonstrate that it has a degree of research credibility through stated supervision arrangements.
- In order to be convincing, supervisors should have training and expertise in the kind of research work they are supervising.
- Given that mental health care is a complex multi-professional endeavour, research in health services often benefits from the involvement of a mixed group of professionals.
- Insights from other professions such as nursing and psychology can strengthen the design and methodology of research conducted by psychiatrists. Multi-professional and multi-agency research is more complex to deliver but can be ultimately more rewarding to the researcher and more valid for the report reader.

It is worth considering in any team of researchers the ways in which various research skills are to be provided. It is unlikely, for example, that any one person can have the depth of knowledge to cover adequately diverse elements such as methodology, statistics and health economics. Furthermore, researchers who forget that successful research needs hands-on practical implementation will soon run into trouble if their teams consist of only theoretical strategists! In summary:

- Researchers must be adequately trained and be perceived as competent.
- The team may be required to demonstrate this competence.
- Multi-disciplinary research work may be difficult but has a number of benefits.
- Research requires practical implementation and this includes intermittent checks that progress is being maintained.

PAST AND CURRENT RESEARCH KNOWLEDGE

There are a number of ways in which evaluation can be undertaken, including:

- Research.
- Audit.
- Service development.
- Various quality initiatives.

One of the features of research which distinguishes it from other types of investigation is that the work should lead to new (generalizable) knowledge. Those wishing to carry out research must, therefore, first explore the existing evidence base including published literature, in the form of:

- Books.
- Journal articles.
- Reports.
- Other widely available dissemination material.

This provides access to a large proportion of the evidence base. The technical advances and availability of CD-ROM and on-line literature search facilities also mean that this section is now the most easily accessible. The techniques and strategies for performing a systematic search of this evidence are explored in Chapter 4.

A second broad category of evidence is known as the 'grey literature'. This term refers to reports and reviews which have not been widely circulated – typically:

- Organizational 'in house' reports.
- Academic dissertations.
- Local and professional newsletters.
- Conference posters.

The most difficult, but arguably the most important area to consider is other current research. Details of current funded research can often be obtained from:

- Non-commercial funding bodies (e.g. Medical Research Council (MRC), Association of Medical Research Charities (AMRC) etc.).
- NHS Regions.
- Commercial research sponsors (e.g. pharmaceutical companies).

Direct contact with any funders appropriate to your research area should be made, particularly if you are seeking grant funding for your project. Again the rapid development of information technology is a real bonus to researchers – many larger funding bodies maintain web-sites, while the NHS sponsored *National Research Register* (NRR) details current research funded by the NHS and major charities. To find out more, contact: Mr Sam Brown, NHS Executive RDD, Room GW59, Quarry House, Quarry Hill, Leeds LS2 7UE.

Finally, prospective researchers should find out what is going on locally. Most organizations which foster research have dedicated research support units (for example, Research and Development (R&D) departments in the NHS) which maintain administrative details of current research activity.

CHOOSING A METHODOLOGY

This chapter and book cannot provide an exhaustive guide to the wide variety of different research methodologies and readers are directed towards specialist texts. However, a broad distinction can be made between *quantitative* and *qualitative* methods which themselves derive from positivist and naturalist philosophies of science.

Positivist (quantitative) methodologies

The term 'positivism' is usually attributed to the philosopher Comte in the nineteenth century. It is associated with four basic beliefs, summarized by von Wright:[2]

- Researchers should be objective, impartial and neutral observers of environmental phenomena.
- 'Fact' is an absolute concept unaffected by the impact of the researcher or the research method.
- There is a unity of scientific method which can be applied to any subject under investigation and that this method, developed from the natural sciences, defines the methodological standard by which all scientific endeavours can be judged.
- Natural laws exist and as such, 'cause and effect' relationships can be discovered wherever they are sought, providing that the methodologies are robust enough.

Positivism became associated with certain methodological developments which are widely used in all branches of science. Chief amongst these is the experiment:

- The idea of experimental manipulation of discrete variables stems from the belief in cause and effect referred to earlier.
- If parts of the environment under investigation can be manipulated in certain ways a process of deductive reasoning can be used to discover scientific laws which predict outcomes and are generalizable to other comparable situations.
- This is the essence of sciences such as physics and chemistry. It is also the major way in which medical science has been conceptualized during the rapid growth in medical research over the last 50 years.

At the peak of positivistic methodological development in health research is the *randomized controlled trial* (RCT). Here:

- An intervention is being tested (a new drug for example) and the researchers randomly allocate research subjects to different experimental conditions, each condition quite separate, usually involving a comparison between an active drug and an inert compound called a placebo.
- A non-intervention condition (maybe a waiting list) might be used as an additional comparison group.
- Assessments of research subjects are made by measuring the target dependent variables before and after the intervention by researchers who are 'blind' to the experimental condition.
- This procedure measures the effects of the intervention which are then compared with the other conditions.
- Terms such as *independent variable* – the antecedent condition manipulated by the experimenter (e.g. drug level) – and *dependent variable* – the variable used to measure the effect of the independent variable (e.g. memory test score) – are used.
- Finally, statistical tests are applied to check the *validity* and *reliability* of the findings against the possibility that they may have occurred by chance and to determine whether the predictions made by the experimenter have borne fruit.

Naturalistic (qualitative) methodologies

Naturalism, of which ethnography and anthropology are two examples, stems from a hermeneutic philosophical tradition and rejects the positivist's view of science. Positivism leads scientists to manipulate the world, a method which naturalists reject as leading to an essentially false representation of what is really happening, particularly when positivist researchers apply their methods to the complex social worlds of human beings. Researchers using naturalist approaches:

- Try to understand the meaning of events within a natural setting.
- Try to understand research subjects' own understandings of their experience and apply these to the particular context under study.
- Believe that objectivity is just not possible and researchers' own actions will change the situation under investigation.
- Believe that the values of the researcher will influence the conduct of the experiment and the analysis of the data.

This latter point has been most clearly articulated by feminist researchers, many of whom[3] reject the positivist research tradition, its associated methodologies and techniques because they represent scientific paradigms bound up in a male vision of the world. Jayaratne[4] describes feminist objections to traditional research in the social sciences in the following way:

- Traditional research supports sexist and elitist values.
- Relevant research is under-utilized.
- Exploitative relationships exist among research staff.
- Research 'subjects' are often deceived and manipulated for the purposes of the research study.
- Methodological rigour is actually frequently overlooked when expedient.
- Quantitative research does not convey a true understanding of the persons under study.

Perhaps the clearest distinction between positivist and naturalist traditions is in the development of theory:

- Positivist science is hypothetico-deductive in that pre-defined theories direct the process of data collection whereas
- Naturalistic research methods often start with observation – unstructured initially – and from this develop theories by a process of induction, moving from data towards generalizations, hypotheses and theory.

The most influential of these methods has probably been the work of Glaser and Strauss,[5] who coined the term 'grounded theory'. This is a creative exercise in examination of data which explicitly uses the researcher's own intellectual powers of interpretation to fit the data into categories provided by the data themselves, not imposed by the researcher's own pre-defined groups. Rigour is maintained by the requirement that data should fit the categories at high and low levels.

Choosing the research method to be used

The two traditions described above have often been simplistically identified with

- Quantitative (numerical, deductive, experimental, statistical) and
- Qualitative (descriptive, inductive, observational) research methods.

In the debate between naturalistic and positivistic ideas, some writers[6] have suggested that philosophical considerations are so important that researchers face a dichotomous choice between the two methods. Others[7,8] have argued that methodological pluralism is the better approach and that some research questions are better answered with qualitative methods, other questions best addressed through quantitative research.

Increasingly, the term 'process evaluation' is being used to describe research (whether the primary research is being conducted in a qualitative or quantitative manner) which gives insight into *what* is going on and *why* people are behaving the way they are.[9] Qualitative methods are particularly suitable for this purpose, adding much to quantitative research data frameworks. Process evaluation can add meaning and depth to outcome studies.

In health and related research, methodological pluralism is being urged ever more strongly by workers such as Nick Black[10] and Roger Jones.[11] The view is increasingly being taken that a mixture of both types of research techniques will answer more completely the questions being addressed by today's health services researchers. The addition of qualitative methods to the prevailing quantitative research culture will, it is argued:

- Enhance research by clarifying how data are defined from quantitative research.
- Provide questions to be asked.
- Generate theories to be tested.
- Explain unexpected quantitative results.
- Provide illuminative insights into data gathered by more conventional quantitative methods.

New researchers are, therefore, encouraged to explore a range of methodological options (Table 3.1). Simplistic adherence to exclusively quantitative or qualitative methods may limit the utility of research results. The key question should be, 'How will my research question best be answered?'

Table 3.1 *Research methods*

Experiments	The experiment is the manipulation of discrete *independent* variables in order to see what impact this manipulation has on *dependent* variables, for example morbidity, length of stay in hospital etc.
Randomized controlled trial (RCT)	Random allocation to alternative preventive, therapeutic or diagnostic interventions with follow up to determine the effect of the interventions compared to the alternatives (which might include no intervention).
Crossover trial	A similar comparative study to an RCT but where two interventions are switched after a specified period of time to measure the impact of each intervention on the same individuals.
Quasi-experimental designs	Comparative trials which are not randomized but pragmatic comparisons of interventions within the same group or between groups; examples include, controlled before and after studies, interrupted time series and switch back designs.
Single case experimental designs	Similar to quasi-experimental designs but involving single case comparisons where interventions in a single case are sequentially implemented and sometimes withdrawn compared to baseline data.

▶

Surveys	Surveys provide a description of a sample of a population by collection of quantifiable data followed by examination and analysis of those data in order to discover patterns and correlations between variables.
Cohort samples	Groups of people followed up for a specified period on a repeated basis, the groups of people usually having common characteristics (e.g. smokers).
Case control studies	A retrospective analysis of factors thought to influence, for example the health of a cohort of patients. Case control studies start with a disorder and look backwards over time to discover factors which may have caused the disorder (e.g. patients with anxiety disorders exposure to previous stressful life events).
Other surveys	Many other types of surveys exist differentiated by the types of sampling (e.g. stratification, matching, quota etc.).
Naturalistic approaches	Naturalistic methodologies emphasize the understanding of the meaning of the event within the natural setting from the subject's point of view. They involve no manipulation of variables and no assumption of cause and effect. Qualitative research does not use statistical or random sampling, rather subjects are chosen in a purposive or theoretical way to add value to the research study.
Observational studies	Participant and non-participant observation of natural settings by a researcher embedding themselves in the 'field'. The researcher attempts to understand the situation from the perspective of other actors by becoming closely interwoven with the situation. Ethnographic and anthropological analysis techniques predominate.
Focus groups and interviews	Structured, unstructured or open individual and group interviews with research subjects where the researcher analyses the interview transcripts to understand the nature of the subjects' experiences.

REVIEWING THE QUALITY OF THE PROJECT

When the project is being developed, it is usual for the detail to be subject to revision as different stakeholders (researchers, supervisor, statistician, managers etc.) are given the chance to contribute to it. This process helps to improve the quality of the project, but is not necessarily very objective, as the stakeholders, by definition, are intimately involved with it. There are three points in the project's life-span when it is likely to be reviewed by people other than the stakeholders.

1. Independent peer review

It is usual for valid research to have been through an independent peer review process. This involves at least one independent expert reviewing the project proposal in order to make recommendations about its:

- Relevance.
- Quality.
- Viability.
- The team's credibility in the research area.

An independent peer review typically occurs when funding is applied for and is organized by the grant-giving body. After submitting your application, you will be told that the project has been rejected, accepted, or will be reconsidered after a number of suggested revisions have been made.

2. Ethics approval

- The Local Ethics Comittee make a judgement about whether or not to allow researchers to recruit 'living subjects' for their research project. While the main focus of this review is to ensure that it does patients no harm (see Chapter 12), it would clearly be unethical to allow subjects to be recruited for a project which lacked:
  - Relevance.
  - Rigor.
  - Was likely to fail for some other reason.

  In other words, the intrinsic quality of the project is also being judged in an ethical review.

3. Final report and resulting journal articles

All dissemination material emanating from the project will be judged by those targeted by it. The reputation of the researchers, anyone associated with the project and the organization(s) sponsoring the project will be at stake. More formally, any article submitted to a peer-reviewed journal will be scrutinized by one or more experts in the field, who advise the editorial board whether to accept, reject or ask for revisions to the submitted article.

It is probable, therefore, that your work will be assessed several times during its development, and many more times once it is complete. Bearing this in mind, and also your professional responsibility to research participants, colleagues and sponsoring organization(s), it is both unethical and unprofessional to start a research study which is poorly designed or unlikely to answer the research question adequately. Interestingly, a survey of 164 funding institutions identified the following top three reasons for project rejection:[12]

- Insignificant problem.
- Poorly defined resources.
- Unclear what problem is being addressed.

The process of getting funding is vital to the project's success, but the *critique mentality* should be a constant theme to the research team over the duration of the project. Projects should be defensible against the following points at least:

- Is it clear why the research is necessary?
- Will the findings be generalizable?
- Is the supporting literature review comprehensive?
- Is the method appropriate to the research question?
- Are the outcome measures appropriate?
- Are the views and experiences of the subjects/participants an integral part of the research?
- How is researcher bias being addressed?
- Are appropriate statistical tests being used – do they have the power to pick up the differences/relationships predicted?
- Can the required subject numbers be recruited in the time-scale?
- Does the research team have the necessary experience/expertise to carry out the research?

RESOURCES AND COSTS

A *resource* is anything which is used in the course of the research project. This includes researchers' time, supplies and equipment, services, excess costs of treatment and overheads. *Costs* are the financial values associated with each resource.

There are four key points to bear in mind:

- Do not underestimate the costs of research.
- Are the costs worked out by the finance department appropriate to your organization (e.g. a university research support unit)?
- Follow the guidelines for any funding bodies you are applying to.
- When writing a proposal allow for the finance department's time in turning around project costing.

In practice, it is easiest to consider each stage of the project separately, and identify the resources required for each stage. Identify the resources first – let your finance department provide the actual costs of these.

Resources may include:

- Researchers' time.
- Excess costs of treatments (i.e. the costs of any treatment which are greater than the costs of 'standard' treatment).
- Equipment not currently available.
- Equipment which is available – indicate that there is no cost.
- Consumables (e.g. paper, computer disks etc.).
- Special support services (clinical, technical, administrative) required.
- Academic and clinical supervision.
- Copyright fees for questionnaires.
- Administration (phone, fax, post and photocopying).

Attaching costs to the resources

It is the policy of many funding bodies to require signed authorization from the finance department who will be administering the grant. Many organizations also have research policies which require input from their finance department. Given that one or both of these conditions will apply, it is worth making contact at the earliest opportunity with the finance department. Although you may have a fair idea of the costs attached to your resources, a financial expert will ensure that:

- Salary costs take account of both annual increments and 'add on costs' (superannuation and National Insurance).
- Organizational discounts are applied to equipment and consumables (e.g. some research work in universities is VAT free).
- Overheads are calculated appropriately.

Overheads

Some funding bodies allow applicants to claim an amount of money to cover unspecified organization costs – the 'hidden' costs of running the organization – including:

- Finance.
- Personnel.
- Corporate departments.
- Costs of depreciation.
- Insurance.
- Buildings and electrical power.

Where allowable, the overheads are often calculated as a prescribed percentage of the total resource costs, or more commonly as a percentage of the staff costs. It should be noted that overheads are returned to the organization; they do not form part of the research budget and cannot be called upon during the project.

Universities have a different definition and formula for calculating overheads. University overheads are those standing costs of running research support services which used to be allocated directly to universities from the government, but which are now given as part of a standard arrangement with government funding bodies such as the research councils (for example, MRC). Currently the research councils allow 47% of staff costs to be charged as overheads by universities.

ETHICAL ISSUES

The modern requirement for the ethical approval of research involving human subjects stems from the publication of the Nuremberg Code, following the end of the Second World War.[13] Ethical issues must always be considered at an early stage in the development of a research project. Ethics is a complex and specialist field and this area is outlined in greater detail in Chapter 12. Certain broad principles should guide all researchers:

- The project should do no harm.
- Participants should be able to give sufficiently informed and free consent to their recruitment into and continuing participation in the research and should be able to refuse to participate at any stage without compromising their rights to any health care they require.
- Participants' confidentiality will be protected and data security will be sufficiently apparent to them.
- The project should not make unethically heavy demands of participants (i.e. it should not exploit them).
- The project should give something back to research participants.

A research protocol should specify any ethical issues raised by the research and how these will be addressed including, where appropriate, submission to a local or multicentre Ethics Committee.

Consent

Anyone entering a research programme as a participant, subject or respondent:

- Should be given a full description of that programme.
- Should not be required to do anything or give out any information unless they have fully understood the purpose of the study.
- Should agree to procedures contained within it.
- Should be given accurate, truthful and easily understood information about the study.

Only then can they give informed consent.

Furthermore, non-participation or initial participation and then subsequent withdrawal from the study should not prejudice their right to any services which are associated with the study.

It is common for patients or research participants to be given an information leaflet which clearly spells out:

- The purpose of the research.
- That information collected is *only* to be used for the research purpose.
- That the results of the research are confidential.
- That connections between data and patient names will be destroyed after data coding.
- That patients have an absolute right not to participate in the research, may withdraw their consent at any time and that by doing so they will not prejudice their right to receive any health care they require.
- A space for their signature to indicate they have read, understood and agreed to the information above.

Confidentiality

It is the responsibility of all professionals, whether engaged in research or not, to maintain the confidentiality of any individual for whom they hold information. In practice, it is required that researchers take active steps to preserve confidentiality, so that it would be impossible for unauthorized people to be able to attribute data to a particular individual. There are many different methods of research, from qualitative through to quantitative, employing very different data collection and analysis, but researchers must ensure that, whatever methodology they follow, the confidentiality of individuals is of paramount importance, and must be preserved. The maintenance of confidentiality is protected by legislation, including the Data Protection Act (1984). The Data Protection Act[14] encompasses eight principles:

- Data should be obtained lawfully.
- Personal data may only be held for the purpose specified.
- Personal data shall not be disclosed.
- Personal data held shall be adequate, relevant and not excessive in relation to the stated purpose.
- Personal data shall be accurate.
- Personal data shall not be kept any longer than is necessary for the specified purpose.
- An individual is entitled to know whether there are data held for which that individual is the subject, and if so, to access that data, and correct or erase it.
- Personal data shall be held securely, to prevent unauthorized access, alteration, disclosure or destruction, or accidental loss.

Databases which include personal information are required to be registered under the 1984 Data Protection Act. Practical steps to preserve the confidentiality of subjects also include the appropriate storage of data and the use of scrambling techniques for electronic data (for example electronic encryption and password protection). A beneficial spin off is that data are unlikely to be lost, stolen, altered or accidentally damaged (e.g. by hot coffee) if it is kept in a locked cabinet and only removed when actively in use.

Exploitation and participation

Another important issue to be considered is to address the concerns of many that research should not exploit those who are often called 'subjects'. Traditionally, the positivistic research perspective sees a clear dividing line between researchers and 'subjects', where subjects are the items of study and have no rights to feedback on the data they provide for the researchers to study. It is distasteful to many that some researchers consider that they have no more moral obligation to share research information with human participants than non-human subjects.[3, 15, 16] These authors have argued that it is more equitable to regard 'subjects' as research participants with a reciprocal right to the personal and grouped information their data provide.

- Researchers should consider the burden which collecting their data places on research participants. Of particular importance are the effects of extra invasive tests – physical or psychological – and any stressful impact this may have on participants.
- Researchers should always be mindful of the difference in power between themselves and research participants in any relationship with patients and should not use this to impose excessive burdens on research participants.
- Where and whenever possible, people who give of their time and information should be given any summary and interpretative information gleaned from the data personal to them together with overall summary information about the results of the research project itself.

Other ethical issues

There are many specific examples of ethical dilemmas which this introductory text cannot consider. Some examples include:

- When designing controlled trials researchers have to address the difficult issue of withholding the experimental treatment from control groups when the efficacy of this treatment has already been demonstrated in pilot work and becomes increasingly evident throughout the trial.
- In rapidly developing fields 'treatment as usual' – a common comparison condition – may itself change.
- How long should the control group be denied the experimental treatment intervention after they have finished the 'treatment as usual' condition?

For discussions of these and other ethical dilemmas the reader is directed to specialist texts.

PROJECT MANAGEMENT

Any successful piece of work, including research, must be well planned and managed to ensure that it progresses as planned. Project management should be realized through:

- The use of a series of explicitly and unambiguously defined tasks.
- Individual responsibilities.
- Deadlines.

There are two major perspectives; that of those undertaking the project and that of the wider group of stakeholders in the project. The former require highly detailed practical plans, which are defined in an *Action plan*.

The stakeholders are usually more interested in an overview of the project's progress, and in the periodic deliverables, or outcomes of the project as it progresses. The *Research outcome management system* is a mechanism which facilitates this process.

Action plan

- The action plan is the highly detailed planning required for the day-to-day operation of the project.
- It is overseen by the Project Steering Group, who are responsible for ensuring that the project runs smoothly from start to finish. This group must agree a set of progress meetings throughout the project's life, and these should be minuted.
- The lead researcher is responsible for chairing these meetings, and for chasing up any member who fails to attend without good reason.
- Although it is tempting to embed the action plan in the minutes, it is greatly preferable for this to exist as a separate document which should be amended after each meeting as required. The minutes serve as an historic record of the reasons behind any changes.

The action plan should dissect the project protocol, breaking it down into a number of tasks. Each task should have a start date and finish date, and be the responsibility of a single named individual. The following should not be forgotten:

- Definition of the roles of each researcher in relation to the protocol.
- Periodic monitoring arrangements.
- Arrangements for approval – ethics, indemnity, organizational permission etc. Note that there is a lead time for each of these, which cannot be overlooked.

- Liaison with the finance department administering the project. (Again allow for lead time.)
- Acquisition of equipment, consumables, project staff. This could take longer than expected and significantly delay the project. Plan ahead.
- Patient/participant recruitment.
- Data collection and storage. Electronic data should be periodically backed up, and an off-site copy maintained (in case of fire, flood, theft etc.).
- Communication with stakeholders.
- Dissemination.

Research outcome management

All too often, research projects start off with high expectations only to flounder due to unforeseen difficulties, such as difficulty recruiting research participants. Worse still, many research teams plough on without realizing problems are looming and time is running out. It is a sadly neglected but vital aspect of any research project to have a rigorous system of project management built into the research process.

All research projects have outcomes which result from different stages of the project. Obvious examples are the paper based ones, including:

- Protocol.
- Ethics form.
- Grant application.
- Participant recruitment letter.
- Progress report.
- Article for publication.
- Final report.

Note that these are mostly generated either at the beginning of the project, or towards the end. Other, less obvious deliverables associated with the progress of the project over the lengthier middle stages can be constructed from the protocol. These could be:

- The recruitment of the first/next 40 participants.
- The rating of the first/next 20 questionnaire scales.
- Data entry of the first/next 100 records onto computer.

Equally, each project has identifiable stages, such as:

- Data analysis.
- Writing up.
- Dissemination.

These are likely to *overlap*. In addition:

- Each stage has a start date and finish date, the latter often referred to as a milestone.

- It is possible to combine the deliverables and milestones into a practical set of research outcomes.

The research outcomes define the detailed progress of the project, and inform the stakeholders of exactly what is happening, and what needs to happen. It allows problems to be addressed at the time they arise, rather than at the supposed end of the project, by which time it is usually too late. We suggest that project teams review their progress against these overlapping outcomes at least quarterly. An example of how information is likely to flow in a research outcome management system for an 18-month project with 100 research participants is summarized in Table 3.2.

Table 3.2 *An example of how information might flow in a hypothetical research outcome management system involving 100 subjects*

	1st quarter	**2nd quarter**	**3rd quarter**	**4th quarter**	**5th quarter**	**6th quarter**
Seek ethical approval	✓					
Ethical approval given		✓				
Patient recruitment (numbers)		20	40	40		
Treatment phase (numbers)		10	30	40	20	
Data analysis (total numbers)				50 (half the data)		100 (all the data)
Dissemination				Interim project report		Final project report

By reviewing the progress of the project in this manner, the complex and overlapping milestone deliverables can be monitored and problems identified and addressed at an early stage before they become a serious threat to the viability of the project.

DISSEMINATION

Dissemination is the production of material by which the results of research are imparted to others including:

- Subject/participants.
- Research collaborators.
- Colleagues.
- Professional bodies.
- Managers.
- Media.
- The general public.

Dissemination is arguably the most important aspect of research. As Day[17] points out, ideas and discoveries only become useful when they are publicized. A more detailed account of how to go about publishing your findings is found in Chapter 11. The process should naturally occur after an event or series of events, but is often overlooked. Researchers can be research-weary at the end of a long project, or just too modest to show their work to peers and others, and it is possible for the production of dissemination materials to be forgotten. Remember though, that researchers have a responsibility to stakeholders to disseminate research findings.

All research protocols should include a specific plan on how the research results will be disseminated and how any recommendations arising from it will be communicated within the stakeholders and to a wider audience:

- Who are the target audiences?
- Which method is best at reaching each target audience?
- What should the content be in each case?
- Have you allowed time in the project plan for producing and presenting dissemination material; are there any resource issues?

Dissemination of material

However the research is disseminated, the material produced should be well structured. A framework is a useful starting point, and the IMRD model (introduction, method, results and discussion) has stood the test of time well.[18] In addition:

- The use of dry scientific language in articles is not necessary to indicate academic quality.[19]
- Researchers should strive to avoid technical and scientific phrases which may alienate their target audiences.
- Jargon, defined as being the opposite of plain English,[20] should also be avoided.
- It is always worth considering innovative methods of dissemination such as stakeholder workshops, seminars or other local media.

Whilst the next section deals mainly with academic writing, a larger or more relevant audience will usually be reached through local events or more 'journalistic' media.

Submission for publication

Journals and other publications which accept articles from researchers each have their own requirements for submitted articles.

- Many of the large circulation peer reviewed and professional journals publish guidelines as an integral part of the journal.
- For those which do not, and for local and organizational newsletter type publications, contact the editor and ask what the requirements are.
- It is necessary for researchers to meet these publication guidelines; articles will not be considered unless they do.

There are, however, two more fundamental responsibilities for researchers concerning publication. The lead researcher must:

- Determine who is eligible to be an author.
- Circulate each draft to all named authors to ensure consensus prior to submission.

The BMJ's guidelines for publication has a section on authorship[21] and in the absence of any other such official guidance, these should be adhered to. They state that:

> 'authorship credit should be based only on substantial contribution to a) conception and design, or analysis and interpretation of data; and to b) drafting the article or revising it critically for important intellectual content; and on c) final approval of the version to be published.'

Authors should therefore be aware that:

- Each author is responsible for the accuracy of the article.
- Each revision must be circulated by the nominated 'contact for correspondence' and approved by all co-authors.
- The printed article should be circulated to each of the co-authors.
- In order to facilitate the dissemination of both the specific project, and the wider need to increase awareness of evidence-based practice, copies of the article should also be distributed to any units or clinics where the research took place, to any appropriate internal libraries or information centres, and to the R&D departments of organizational stakeholders.

Before submitting an article, therefore:

- Check that it meets the publisher's guidelines.
- Use all the electronic tools available, such as spelling and grammar checker and 'readability' analyser.
- Circulate the draft copies to all stakeholders for comment.

On acceptance for publication, researchers must:

- Circulate any proof copies to each author for approval.
- Ensure that copies of the published article are distributed to all named authors.

KEY POINTS

- The research questions: these should be clear, precise and use simple language. They lead on to the research method and can be written in a qualitative 'grand tour with subquestions' format or as positivistic hypotheses.
- Stakeholders: these include researchers, organizations, research subjects/participants and funders. Their views need balancing but add richness and validity to any research project.
- The project team: a project team should consist of individuals with different and complementary skills. Multi-disciplinary teams enrich most health care research.
- Past and current research knowledge: knowledge of the evidence base in any field can be found through published literature, grey literature and indices of current research.
- Choosing a methodology: naturalistic and positivistic philosophies lead to different research methods. Within each tradition there are huge choices of methodology but the method chosen should be one which is likely to answer the research questions. Methodological pluralism can often be more effective in researching the complete picture.
- Reviewing the quality of the project: stakeholders in a project steering group can improve the quality of a project but independent peer review, ethical approval and submission for publication are specific opportunities for project or results scrutiny.
- Resources and costs: all research is costly and costs should be assessed by financial experts with the research team leaving enough time for this process to be completed accurately.
- Ethical issues: projects should do no harm, pay attention to consent and confidentiality, not make unethically heavy demands on research subjects/participants and should try to give something back to those people or organizations who have been researched.
- Project management: well-managed projects need an action plan which assigns roles and responsibilities to the project team. Research outcome management can assist in ensuring milestone deliverables are met.

▶

- Dissemination: research which is not disseminated effectively and widely is a waste of effort. Local, regional and national media should be employed and methods other than peer reviewed journals are essential.

REFERENCES

1. Creswell, J. W. *Research Design – Qualitative and Quantitative Approaches*. 1994; Sage Publishing, California.
2. Von Wright, G. H. *Explanation and Understanding*. 1971; Routledge, London.
3. Oakley, A. Sexism in official statistics. In: *Demystifying Social Statistics* (Irvine, J., Miles, I., Evans, J. eds). 1979; Pluto, London.
4. Jayaratne, T. E. The value of quantitative methodology for feminist research. In: *Theories for Women's Studies* (Bowles, G., Klein, R. D. eds). 1983; Routledge and Kegan Paul, London.
5. Glaser, B., Strauss, A. *The Discovery of Grounded Theory; Strategies for Qualitative Research*. 1967; Aldine, Chicago.
6. Porter, M. 'Second-hand ethnography': some problems in analysing a feminist project. In: *Analysing Qualitative Data* (Bryman, A., Burgess, R. G. eds). 1994; Routledge, London.
7. Abell, P. Methodological achievements in sociology over the past few decades with special reference to the interplay of qualitative and quantitative methods. In: *What has Sociology Achieved?* (Bryant, C., Becker, H. eds). 1990; Macmillan, London.
8. Bryman, A. Quantitative and qualitative research; further reflections on their integration. In: *Mixing Methods; Qualitative and Quantitative Research*, (Brannen, J. ed.). 1992; Avebury, Aldershot.
9. Tones, B. K., Tilford, S. *Health Education; Effectiveness, Efficiency and Equity*. 1994; Chapman Hall, London.
10. Black, N. Editorial. Why we need qualitative research. *Journal of Epidemiology and Community Health*, 1994; **48**, 425–26.
11. Jones, R. Why do qualitative research? *British Medical Journal*. 1995; **311**, 2.
12. Coley, S. M., Scheinberg, C. A. *Proposal Writing*. 1990; Sage Publishing, California, p.37.
13. Royal College of Physicians of London *Research Involving Patients*. 1990; RCPoL, London.
14. The Data Protection Registrar *Guidelines to the Data Protection Act 1984*. 1994; Wilmslow, Office of the Data Protection Registrar.
15. Frieze, I. H., Parsons, J. E., Johnson, P. B., Ruble, D. N., Zellman, G. L. *Women and Sex Roles; A Social Psychological Perspective*. 1978; Norton, New York.

16. Morgan, D. *Doing Feminist Research*. 1981; Routledge and Kegan Paul, London.
17. Day, A. *How to Get Research Published in Journals*. 1996; Gower Publishing Limited, Aldershot.
18. Jones, R. Disseminating new knowledge to other researchers. In: *Disseminating Research/Changing Practice* (Dunn, E., Norton, P., Stewart, M., Tudiver, F., Bass, M. eds). 1994; Sage Publications, California.
19. McMillan, I. *Effective Writing Skills for Nurses*. 1997; Macmillan Magazines Limited, London.
20. Collinson, D., Kirkup, G., Kyd, R., Slocombe, L. *Plain English*. 1995; Open University Press, Buckingham.
21. British Medical Journal *Getting published in the BMJ: advice for authors*. 1996; British Medical Journal, **314**, 66–8.

Chapter Four

Carrying out the literature search

Julie Glanville

INTRODUCTION

This chapter explores the process of carrying out a literature review and describes:

1. The purpose of a literature review.
2. Defining the research question and estimating the budget for a review.
3. Identifying resources needed to answer the research question.
4. How to construct search strategies to find research publications relevant to the research question.
5. How to carry out literature searches.
6. How to store the results.
7. Data analysis and synthesis.
8. Documenting the search.

THE PURPOSE OF A LITERATURE REVIEW

Literature reviews are carried out to establish the current state of research knowledge on a given topic, so that subsequent primary research can be based on a sound knowledge base. Increasingly literature reviews, carried out in a systematic way, are becoming a key research methodology providing evidence of effectiveness for practice and policy making:

> 'Decision makers of various types are inundated with unmanageable amounts of information. They have a great need for systematic reviews that separate the known from the unknown and that save them from the position of knowing less than has been proved.'[1]

Literature reviews are conducted to avoid duplication of research and to identify where the needs for future research lie. Whatever the purpose and scope of the literature review it can benefit from the new emphasis on a systematic approach to conducting reviews of clinical effectiveness.[2,3,4] This approach in identifying and gathering data for a review involves:

- Defining a clear research question and criteria for inclusion/selection of studies.
- Identifying the databases and other sources to be searched.
- Preparing comprehensive search strategies.
- Recording the progress of the searches conducted.
- Documenting the searches.

The systematic approach is intended to reduce bias and to encourage the production of an objective and replicable piece of work. Clear planning of the literature review is vital to ensure that the researcher and any funder have a clear awareness of the resource implications of the work to be undertaken. Even well-focused questions can generate a significant amount of literature to review and assess, which emphasizes the need to plan the review process thoroughly.

This chapter focuses on how to develop a clear question to research and on the literature searching aspects of conducting a literature review. The literature search is just part of the process of conducting a literature review. Reviews may be small-scale or large-scale. Detailed guidance on the whole process of doing large-scale systematic reviews is available from the NHS Centre for Reviews and Dissemination and the Cochrane Collaboration.[3,5] Although many literature reviews, such as those undertaken at the start of a thesis, may not be resourced to the scale of systematic reviews, the approaches used in systematic reviews, such as protocol design, clear inclusion and exclusion criteria, data collection, and study combination, can be drawn on to inform the production of smaller scale reviews. The process of undertaking a systematic review is summarized in Table 4.1.

Table 4.1 *Phases in undertaking a systematic review*

Phase 0	Identification of the need for a review.
Phase 1	Background research and problem specification.
Phase 2	Requirements for the review protocol.
Phase 3	Literature searching and study retrieval.
Phase 4	Assessment of studies for inclusion on the basis of relevance and design.
Phase 5	Assessing the validity of studies.
Phase 6	Data extraction.
Phase 7	Data synthesis.
Phase 8	Structure of the report.
Phase 9	Peer review: scientific quality, content and relevance.
Phase 10	Submission of report and plans for dissemination.

Modified from[3]

DEFINING THE RESEARCH QUESTION AND BUDGET ISSUES

The first stage of a literature review is to set the parameters of the review by clearly defining the research question. The research question may begin as a vague idea but must be refined into a clear statement of the research question to be answered. Rather than a broad question such as 'do antidepressants work?', it is better to be as focused as possible, for example, 'are new (and expensive) antidepressants (such as SSRIs) any more effective or better tolerated than older (tricyclic) antidepressants?'. This question is much easier to research and could itself be further refined in terms of population groups and other factors.

To refine a broad topic, it can be helpful to consider the following issues:

- What is the intervention or interventions under investigation?
- What is the population of interest?
- What is the setting, for example, outpatient or inpatient?
- What outcomes are of interest?
- What study designs are important to this research?

Some of these issues may need to be clarified by a brief initial search of relevant databases in order to assess the volume of literature that may be available. Other questions which may help in the definition of the question and limit the search include:

- Date limits – if the technology was only recently introduced, searching can be limited to more recent years, thus saving time and money.
- Geographic limits – if the intervention or setting are oriented within the UK it may be decided only to search for UK studies. Similarly it may be possible to exclude explicitly certain geographical areas such as developing countries.
- Language – if no translation facilities are available or there is no budget for translation, it may not be deemed essential to search for non-English language papers.
- Non-journal articles – if there are other publications formats where relevant studies may appear such as conference papers, or dissertations, then databases which cover these formats need to be identified.

Defining these limits can often make searching easier. Decisions on some of the limits will be determined by the research budget: the more databases searched, the more expensive the search process. In addition, the more documents identified by searches, the more inter-library loans will tend to be required. Limits are also affected by the time available for carrying out the literature review. If only two months are available, clearly the review will be less ambitious than if a whole year is available, as is typical for a full scale systematic review. The important thing is to be explicit about the extent of the literature review and to document the decisions which define the scope of the review.

The budget

Literature reviews, particularly systematic reviews, can be very expensive to produce, and it is vital to know the level of available resources before planning extensive searches. Depending on the resources of local libraries and the level of workplace support, some or all of the following costs may fall on a prospective literature reviewer:

- The costs of searching on-line databases. Some databases, such as MEDLINE, are widely available free of charge in medical libraries. Others, such as EMBASE (Excerpta Medica) or PsycLIT may incur a charge. These costs can often be hard to estimate and will depend upon the subject and extent of the search. A health or medical librarian will be able to advise on approximate figures once a search question has been clarified.
- The costs of photocopying articles and other material in local libraries.
- The costs of inter-library loans for material not available in local libraries. Health and medical librarians can advise on local charging policies. These charges can be high and may be higher for some types of publication, such as theses.
- The costs of visits to other libraries including travel and photocopying.
- Internet access: many institutions and professional organizations may provide free access to the Internet including the World Wide Web. If free access is not available, personal Internet access software and support facilities can be bought from many suppliers. If searching is carried out at home it will incur telephone charges.
- Bibliographic software to manage references (see later in this chapter).
- Clerical or secretarial help to type in references (see later in this chapter) and manage inter-library loan requests and receipts.
- Fees for advice from specialists, for example some librarians may charge for their time if searches are lengthy, statistical advice may be required at the data synthesis stage, and computing support may be required to set up bibliographic and Internet software.
- Researchers' own time.

IDENTIFYING RESOURCES TO ANSWER THE QUESTION

There may be many potentially relevant information resources which can offer material to help answer the research question. A local medical, health or academic library is a good place to start, because the librarian will be able to discuss what is available locally and what is available elsewhere, and at what cost. The following sections cover the types of resources which can be examined to compile a wish-list of useful resources to search.

Indexes to subject resources

It is often difficult to know where to look for published and unpublished research. There are many guides to information resources and databases that may be good starting points to identify resources to be searched (Table 4.2). As well as paper directories, the World Wide Web (WWW) offers many subject-specific sites where searchers are offered a range of services and links to other services.[6]

Table 4.2 *Selected guides to information resources*

1. Morton, L. and Godbolt, S. eds. (1992) *Information sources in the medical sciences.* 4th edn. London: Bowker Saur.
2. Kiley, R. (1996) *Medical information on the Internet: a guide for health professionals.* Edinburgh: Churchill Livingstone.
3. Domoney, L., Carmel, M., Sawers, C. (1996) *Directory of health and social services databases.* London: Library Association Publishing.
4. Armstrong, C. J. ed. (1993) *World databases in medicine.* London: Bowker Saur.
5. BUBL Subject tree. http://bubl.ac.uk/link/subjects/
6. OMNI (Organising Medical Networked Information) gateway to biomedical resources. http://www.omni.ac.uk/
7. Cognitive and psychological sciences on the Internet – an index to Internet resources relevant to research in cognitive science and psychology. http://matia.stanford.edu/cogsci.html

Existing reviews

To avoid wasted time and effort it is wise not to begin a review or to bid for funding without checking whether there are existing reviews. Some key sources of published and unpublished reviews include:

- The Cochrane Library. This is a collection of databases, two of which are solely databases of systematic reviews of healthcare interventions. The Cochrane Database of Systematic Reviews contains the full text of reviews produced and updated by the Cochrane Collaboration. The Database of Abstracts of Reviews of Effectiveness, produced by the NHS Centre for Reviews and Dissemination at the University of York, contains structured summaries of quality assessed reviews produced by non-Cochrane researchers. Available on CD-ROM and via the Internet (http://www.update-software.com/ccweb/cochrane/cdsr.htm).
- Best evidence. This contains structured abstracts and commentaries on reviews published in major journals. It is available on CD-ROM from BMJ Publishing.
- MEDLINE is a major database which abstracts the published medical literature. It contains thousands of reviews and there are many

predefined search strategies which can be used to retrieve reviews (see below).
- PsycINFO, PsycLIT and Psychological Abstracts. These three versions of the major abstracting service for psychological publications can also be searched for existing reviews.

Ongoing research

As well as completed research, it is also advisable to check for ongoing research, again in order to avoid duplicating someone else's research in progress. Sources of information on ongoing research include:

- National Research Register. This is a register of research ongoing within the NHS and of interest to the NHS. Copies should be available in health, medical and University libraries. See Chapter 3 for the contact address for further information.
- *Current Research in Britain: Social Sciences; Current Research in Britain: Physical Sciences; and Current Research in Britain: Biological Sciences*, are published by Longman, and are available in book and CD-ROM formats.
- Various databases of conference proceedings are available and are useful because some research is presented at conferences, but never published elsewhere. Access to these databases will usually be via a librarian. Proceedings databases include: *Directory of Published Proceedings* (via the Dialog Corporation host); *Inside Conferences* (via the Dialog Corporation host); *Conference Papers Index* (via the Dialog Corporation host) and *Index to Scientific & Technical Proceedings* (BIDS). For information on the Dialog Corporation and BIDS see later in this chapter.
- The Cochrane Library contains records of Cochrane reviews in progress and gives the review protocol.

It may also be worth searching the WWW using a general search engine such as Lycos, or Alta Vista in order to locate ongoing research mentioned on academic web sites and elsewhere. These engines are also available through a variety of Internet Service providers or may be accessed directly:

- Lycos http://www-uk.lycos.com/
- Alta Vista http://www.altavista.digital.com/
- Muscat http://www.muscat.co.uk/

Published articles

Published journal articles are recorded in a range of large international databases which can be searched using a variety of different search software. The same database may be published in a variety of formats:

CD-ROM, on-line or paper. The same database may also be licensed to different publishers and suppliers, and appear with different search interfaces (for example OVID or SilverPlatter). The way that search features are implemented may also be different between particular search interfaces. The largest databases of interest to psychiatrists are MEDLINE, PsycLIT or PsycINFO, EMBASE and the Cochrane Library (Table 4.3).

Table 4.3 *Selected major databases recording journal articles*

PsycLIT (CD-ROM) or *PsycINFO* (on-line database). These are the database versions of the paper publication *Psychological Abstracts.* Since 1967 the database has been recording the international literature in psychology and related behavioural and social sciences, and has indexed publications beyond the journal literature.

MEDLINE is a major source of published biomedical literature, produced by the National Library of Medicine in the USA. Its coverage is 1966 onwards and it increases by more than 400 000 records each year. Most health and medical libraries will provide free access to this database and it is also available at various free WWW sites including that of the National Library of Medicine (http://www.ncbi.nlm.nih.gov/PubMed/).

EMBASE is another major database of pharmacological and biomedical literature and claims a concentration on European sources and drug-related literature. It tends to be very expensive to search. It is available on CD-ROM and via various on-line suppliers.

The Cochrane Library contains a unique collection of more than 150 000 bibliographic records of randomized controlled trials (RCTs) in the *Cochrane Controlled Trials Register* (CCTR). Although many of the records are also on *MEDLINE and EMBASE, CCTR's* advantage is that it provides a quick and focused way of locating RCTs.

SciSearch and *Social SciSearch* (also available as *ISI Current Contents* databases on the BIDS service). These are multidisciplinary databases indexing journals in the sciences and social sciences.

CINAHL is the major database for nursing literature. It is available free in many health and medical libraries and is also available on the Dialog Corporation Service and via other hosts.

Dissertations

Much research is carried out in order to gain a higher degree, but may never reach publication in journal articles. Therefore, dependent on the topic, it may be useful to search resources such as *Dissertation Abstracts Online*. This will probably only be accessible via a librarian. It covers more than 1.2 million doctoral dissertations and master's theses. Although the majority of the records it contains are for US theses, there is increasing Canadian and European coverage. Another useful source for theses is the *Index to Theses accepted for higher degrees by the Universities of Great Britain and Ireland and the Council of National Academic Awards.* This has been published by Aslib since 1967 and is available in large academic libraries.

Conference proceedings

Databases which record conference proceedings are useful routes into research which never gets published in the other formats. Some key databases have already been listed in the Ongoing Research Section.

Grey literature

Guidelines, reports and working papers will often be ignored by the type of databases described above because of their relatively informal publication format. However, they may be retrieved, to a certain extent, using databases such as:

- DH-Data. This is available on the Dialog Corporation Datastar service and is produced by the English Department of Health. It thus contains records of many non-journal publications and has a strong UK coverage. Access will be primarily via a librarian.
- System for Information on Grey Literature in Europe (SIGLE). This database is available via the British Library's Blaiseline host and will probably need to be searched by a librarian. Since 1983 it has indexed documents which cannot be easily identified through normal bookselling channels and covers all subjects.

Books

Books, which may be reviews or textbooks in the research question area, should not be ignored in the review process. Books may not only be valuable introductions and reviews of a topic, but they can also contain many references which a reviewer will want to follow up. However, books can be quite difficult to retrieve because they do not tend to have abstracts on databases and do not often receive the level of subject indexing that journal articles receive. A number of resources give access to some of the largest catalogues in the world:

- OPAC 97. This service, launched in May 1997, provides free access via the World Wide Web to the catalogues of the major British Library collections. URL: http://opac97.bl.uk/
- Library Open Access Catalogues (OPACs) in Higher Education. This WWW site offers links to British and Irish academic library catalogues. URL: http://www.niss.ac.uk/reference/opacs.html
- World-wide library catalogues via Hytelnet at the University of Cambridge. URL: http://www.cam.ac.uk/Hytelnet/

- Library of Congress. A WWW interface to the Library of Congress catalogues which contain millions of records. URL: http://marvel.loc.gov/

Libraries

For some research topics there may be key research institutes and libraries that should be contacted or visited. For example the Institute for Study of Drug Dependence has a library and information service which would be a key resource for researchers in drug dependence. Most libraries will be able to suggest directories of research institutes and libraries.

Handsearching

For a given research question, there may be key journals which should be searched by hand in a library, even if they are also indexed in major databases. Handsearching can compensate for any inadequacies or inconsistencies in database indexing or database searching. Key journals can be identified by examining frequently occurring journal names in the studies which are being retrieved by searches, and by asking experts in the field.

Experts

Contacting known experts in the chosen field may produce helpful suggestions, further literature and more contacts. However, it is best not to rely on experts alone, and the other methods of study identification are necessary to provide as objective a collection of material as possible.

Using electronic-mail (e-mail) discussion lists can also be a way to find out about research in progress or publications of interest. It is polite when using e-mail discussion lists to state the question very clearly and to describe the information sources already searched. To identify mailing lists try the following sites:

- Medical Matrix. http://www.medmatrix.org/index.asp
- CIC HealthWeb. http://healthweb.org
- Liszt: the mailing list directory. http://www.liszt.com/
- Mailbase list. http://www.mailbase.ac.uk/lists.html
- Discussion lists.http://matia.stanford.edu/cogsci/discuss.html

CARRYING OUT THE SEARCH

Once a set of resources to be searched has been identified, the question defined and any limits established, it is time to develop a search strategy to encapsulate the research question. It can be helpful to design the search strategy for the database which may give the richest yield (such as

MEDLINE or PsycLIT) and then to modify it for other databases taking into account differences of database content, coverage and subject indexing.

The following worked example gives an approach to search strategy design:

Example 1. The question: 'Are antidepressants effective in treating childhood depressive disorders?'

The first step is to separate out the concepts involved in the question:

- **disease or illness?** depressive disorder
- **treatment?** antidepressants
- **treatment group?** children
- **study design (if any)?** randomized controlled trials
- **outcomes** less depression

The next stage is to identify limits to the search:

- **date limits?** assume post–1990
- **geographic limits?** assume none
- **language issues?** assume English language only
- **publication formats?** all

Assuming that the first major database to be searched is MEDLINE, the search can be drafted by identifying relevant *textwords* and *subject headings* for each of the major concepts: disease, treatment, treatment group and study design. Many large databases, including PsycINFO and EMBASE, provide subject indexing terms for each article, which are searchable in addition to the words in the title and abstract. The *subject indexing* is a controlled vocabulary or thesaurus used to ensure that records on the same subject receive the same index terms. For example, one author may refer to 'enuresis' in a paper while another may use the phrase 'bed wetting'. The database indexers would identify that these authors are dealing with the same concept and would assign a 'preferred' index term to both of their articles, which might be ENURESIS.[7] The searcher then needs to identify from the thesaurus relevant to the database (for MEDLINE this would be MeSH – Medical Subject Headings) what the preferred term is, and then use it in the search (Table 4.4). However, although the use of keywords improves the recall of articles, it is not possible to rely on indexing totally, so a certain level of redundancy needs to be built into searches by also using textwords. For example, the antidepressants used to treat depressive disorders may be indexed with very specific headings, perhaps for the drug name, or a broad subject heading, for example ANTIDEPRESSIVE AGENTS.

Table 4.4 *Search features of MEDLINE*

Thesauri, such as MeSH, offer valuable search features which can make searching easier. One of the most useful features of MeSH is the *Explosion* facility. This makes use of the 'tree-like' structure of a thesaurus to enter a single term and pick up all the more specific terms beneath it. For example exploding ANTIDEPRESSIVE AGENTS in one tree picks up all the specific antidepressants listed below.

- Antidepressive agents.
- Benactyzine.
- Citalopram.
- Clorgyline.
- Deanol.
- Iproniazid.
- Isocarboxazid.
- Lithium carbonate.
- Nialamide etc.

Terms and concepts can be identified by reading relevant papers and by conducting initial brief searches using the original key words of the question. This approach should produce other papers which can be examined for other textwords and subject headings which may describe the topic of interest. Identifying synonyms and related terms to the main topic is a particular feature of searching for studies to include in systematic reviews and it is used to maximize the comprehensiveness of the search. This is not necessarily the best approach when faced with a question which needs an answer within an hour, although the previous discussions of question definition and limits can be helpful. Table 4.5 shows an example of the type of textwords and subject headings gathered by methods described above.

The other feature of this example is that it makes use of pre-defined strategies produced by other researchers. The randomized controlled trial (RCT) textwords and subject headings are those identified by researchers in the Cochrane Collaboration as helpful to retrieve RCTs in MEDLINE.[8] There are increasing numbers of strategies available to which relevant subject terms can be added:

- A range of strategies including search strategies to locate RCTs can be found at: http://www.ihs.ox.ac.uk/library/filters.html
- Predefined search strategies to locate systematic reviews on MEDLINE and CINAHL are available at the Web site of the NHS Centre for Reviews and Dissemination:
  http://www.york.ac.uk/inst/crd/search.htm
- A variety of predefined search strategies are available via the PubMED free MEDLINE site. These search strategies have been designed

to focus on papers dealing with therapy, diagnosis, aetiology and prognosis:

- http://www.ncbi.nlm.nih.gov/PubMed/clinical.html

Table 4.5 *Identifying textwords and subject index terms for the key concepts*

	Textwords (i.e. a word in the title, abstract and often the subject headings)	**Medical subject headings (MeSH) terms**
A Depressive disorders	depressive disorder(s) severe()depression major()depression dysthymia	depressive disorder/ dysthymic disorder/ neurasthenia/ depression involutional/
B Antidepressants	Antidepressant(s) Antidepressive$ Tricyclics Fluoxetine Sertraline Bupropion Monoamine oxidase ssri(s) selective serotonin	exp antidepressive agents/ exp monoamine oxidase/ exp serotonin uptake inhibitors/ exp benzamides/
C Children	child(ren) adolescen$ teenage$	exp child/
D RCTs	clinical$ trial$ single blind$ double blind$ treble blind$ triple blind$ mask$ placebo$ random$ control$ prospectiv$ volunteer$	randomized controlled trial randomized controlled trials random allocation/ double-blind method/ single-blind method/ controlled clinical trial.pt. clinical trial.pt. exp clinical trials/ placebos/ research design/ comparative study/ exp evaluation studies/ follow-up studies/ prospective studies/

The search might finally look as follows:

1 (depressive adj disorder$).tw.
2 (severe or major) adj depression.tw.
3 dysthymia.tw.
4 depressive disorder/
5 dysthymic disorder/
6 neurasthenia/
7 depression involutional/
8 or/1–7
9 exp antidepressive agents/
10 antidepressant$.tw.
11 antidepressive$.tw.
12 tricyclics.tw.
13 fluoxetine.tw.
14 sertraline.tw.
15 bupropion.tw.
16 (monoamine adj oxidase).tw.
17 exp monoamine oxidase/
18 exp serotonin uptake inhibitors/
19 (ssri or ssris).tw.
20 (selective adj serotonin).tw.
21 exp benzamides/
22 or/9–21
23 exp child/
24 (child or adolescen$ or teenage$ or children).tw.
25 or/23–24
26 randomized controlled trial.pt.
27 randomized controlled trials/
28 random allocation/
29 double-blind method/
30 single-blind method/
31 controlled clinical trial.pt.
32 clinical trial.pt.
33 exp clinical trials/
34 (clinical$ adj5 trial$).tw.
35 ((singl$ or doubl$ or trebl$ or tripl$) adj5 (blind$ or mask$)).tw.
36 placebos/
37 (placebo$ or random$).tw.
38 research design/
39 comparative study/
40 exp evaluation studies/
41 follow-up studies/
42 prospective studies/
43 (control$ or prospectiv$ or volunteer$).tw.
44 or/26–43
45 8 and 22 and 25 and 44
46 limit 45 to english language

The search symbols used are explained in Table 4.6.

The search is now ready to run on the chosen database. In the above example, a series of MeSH terms and textwords for depressive disorders are combined using the OR operator: or/1–8. The OR operator is a command used to combine sets so that any of the terms specified can be retrieved and it has the effect of broadening a search. Then a series of MeSH terms and textwords for antidepressive drugs are searched and the results combined together into the set 22 (or/9–21). The same happens for terms to retrieve the concept of childhood (set 25) and the study design randomized controlled trials (set 43). The four large sets are then combined using the AND operator to achieve the result set 45 which should contain records that have textwords or keywords from all of the four sets (depression, antidepressants, children and RCTs) AND has the effect of narrowing the search. The resulting set is then limited to English-language articles (set 46).

Table 4.6 *Searching features*

Depending on the search software, various commands and features will be available to make searches more sophisticated. Some typical commands (for the OVID interface) are:

- Truncation: $ is a truncation symbol. It is used to pick up plurals and word variants. For example, 'prospectiv$' will retrieve 'prospective' and 'prospectively'.
- Field searching: .pt. is an example of how to restrict the search to a specific field in the database, in this case the Publication Type field. '/' is the OVID symbol for a MeSH term, e.g. 'random allocation/' tells the software to look for the MeSH term 'random allocation' rather than textwords.
- Explosion: 'exp' is the OVID command to explode a MeSH term (see earlier).
- Adjacency: 'adj' is used to stipulate that search terms should be next to each other, for example, 'substance adj abuse' will only retrieve records where those terms appear as a phrase 'substance abuse'. 'adj' with a number, e.g. 'adj4' indicates that the words to be searched can be up to four words apart. Using 'substance adj4 abuse' would retrieve records with phrases such as 'abuse of a narcotic substance was observed'.
- AND, OR and NOT: search terms and search sets can be combined using the Boolean operators of set theory. AND produces smaller sets, OR is used to broaden a search, and NOT excludes terms or sets which are not required (see example search). NOT should be used with care.

This search can now be translated to search other databases. As well as translating the search terms, the syntax of other search interfaces would need to be taken into account. There are several common interfaces such as OVID and WinSPIRS, but searching a range of databases for a literature review may reveal others. Particular areas where translation is important are:

- Any specific search commands, e.g. 's' (for 'search') needs to prefix the search terms in some systems.
- The truncation operator, (e.g. $, ?, *, #).
- The proximity operator, (e.g. adj, (w), near, with).
- The command to achieve subject heading explosion ('exp' in OVID).
- The format for tags such as publication type, (e.g. pt=clinical trial, clinical trial.pt.).
- The way to achieve date and language limits.

Seeking the help of a librarian can help with the translation complexities of different interfaces. Translating searches may also involve dropping some of the facets of the search. With the example above, it would not be necessary, when searching the Cochrane Controlled Trials Register, to use the RCT facet because that database *only* contains RCTs. When no thesaurus is available with a database, the text words will need to be expanded by the searcher in order to compensate for the lack of thesaurus terms.

SEARCH ISSUES

The resources to be searched may be available in a variety of formats and will require different approaches.

Paper-based resources

Some indexes and abstracts may be only available in book form and may require long and systematic searching by hand. The availability of good indexes will make some resources easier to search. Transcribing references into a database can also be time consuming and it can be useful to budget for clerical help if there is a great deal of manual searching to be carried out.

CD-ROMS

CD-ROMs have the advantage of usually being free at the point of use, but may present problems in use. Some search interfaces are unable to cope with large searches, there may be limits on the number of records which can be printed or downloaded and, with large databases, the search may need to be repeated across several disks. Some of these issues can be resolved by early liaison with a librarian who may suggest solutions or change system defaults to allow larger searches or downloads.

On-line services

These offer a huge range of services on a pay per minute and pay per record basis, but they can prove very expensive and have additional access costs as well as annual subscription charges. For these reasons searching tends to be carried out by trained librarians. It will help the librarian to see a detailed search question, a list of search terms and to know as much as possible about how the search can be limited (such as by date or language) and what has already been searched. There are also some 'supermarket' services or hosts which offer Internet access to a wide range of databases. Such hosts include the Dialog Corporation service (who provide two collections of databases called, currently, Dialog and Datastar) and Ovid. These hosts offer 'pay as you go' searching (rather than the subscription fee approach of CD-ROM and paper publishers) whereby the price of the search is determined by the time spent searching the database and the number of records printed or displayed. *BIDS* is a database host organized for the benefit of the UK academic community and offers access to a range of databases including

SciSearch and Social SciSearch. The databases which are available for searching for free will depend on the purchasing decisions of each academic library.

The World Wide Web (WWW)

Increasingly databases are available to search via the WWW. Some may be free and some may charge. Each will have a different search interface of varying levels of sophistication so that search strategies will need to be adapted for each one. The availability of features such as truncation, proximity searching and thesauri, will need to be investigated using any available on-line help. The trade-off between a free WWW-based database and paying for a potentially more sophisticated and quicker on-line search may need to be considered.

Searching through an intermediary

Some resources and services may only be available via an intermediary such as a librarian. Some libraries will search their specialized databases on request and this may be the best solution if the library is at a distance. Briefing an intermediary on the exact nature of the search is made easier if the preliminary work in this chapter has been carried out.

Storing the results

Before the results start to flow in from searches it is important to plan the format they should appear in (this may be called the print format, the export format or the output format) and how they will be stored. The required output format is usually determined by the software being used to store the records. When preparing a literature review it is best to make use of personal bibliographic software which has some or all of the following features:

- Stores references, allowing rapid access, sorting and deduplication.
- Allows easy searching by single words or words in combination.
- Links into word processing packages for easier final document production.

There are many packages available and some organizations buy site licences for particular ones. Some packages will take input from named databases or database interfaces using prepared filters. Others will require the definition of filters to be written by the user. Where possible request search results in a tagged format and it should be relatively straightforward to import them into the bibliographic software. Specifying a preferred format for results in an electronic form such as ‘text files of tagged records’ should make liaison with any intermediaries doing searches less prone to confusion.

Common bibliographies include:

- Reference Manager and Procite. Both are available from Research Information Systems, Brunel Science Park, Building 1, Brunel University, Uxbridge, UB8 3PQ, Tel. 01895–813544. e-mail: uksales@ris.risinc.com (for Product Information in Europe).
- Idealist. Available from Bekon, Tel: 01625–503756.
- Endnote. Available from Cherwell Scientific Publishing, the Magdalen Centre, Oxford Science Park, Oxford, OX4 4GA. http://www.cherwell.com/endnote and http://www.cherwell.com/support.html.

When designing the database to hold the search results consider what additional information that will need to be added to each record. The database can be used to hold the data resulting from analysis of the studies, and typical fields could include:

- Codes to indicate the source database (e.g. MEDLINE).
- Decision fields (e.g. include or exclude from the review).
- Fields to record whether copies have been ordered/have arrived.
- Coding to reflect the study design (e.g. RCT).
- Fields to record data from the original article (such as sample size, intervention, loss to follow-up, blinding method etc.).

The more detailed and pre-planned the database structure is, the easier the final report generation will become. Recording decisions and coding records makes the process as systematic as possible and keeps the data for the review under control.

DATA ANALYSIS AND SYNTHESIS

As publications are collected, the researcher moves into the next stage of the review which involves the analysis of the data from single studies and their synthesis into an overall statement. The methods of data analysis and synthesis are not the focus of this chapter, but guidance on conducting these parts of reviews is available from the NHS Centre for Reviews and Dissemination and the Cochrane Collaboration.[3,5] Although many literature reviews, such as those prepared for theses, may not be resourced to the scale of systematic reviews, the approaches used in systematic reviews can be drawn on to inform the production of smaller scale reviews. Guidance on how to appraise critically studies is available[9] and for difficult methodological questions there is the Cochrane Methodology Database on the Cochrane Library. The latter is a useful bibliography of articles on the many methodological issues surrounding review production.

DOCUMENTING THE SEARCH

The literature search is often forgotten once the analysis of the data begins. However, the description of the search forms a small but vital part of the final written review (Table 4.7). The search description should include the following details:

- Database name and software.
- Dates searched.
- Any limits.
- An outline of at least one of the search strategies.

Table 4.7 *Documenting the search strategy*

Basic requirements:

- Database name.
- Date coverage.
- Host or software version.
- Listing of search terms.

Example:

MEDLINE (OVID CD-ROM interface) 1990–Aug. 1997. Search strategy:

1 (depressive adj disorder$).tw.
2 depressive disorder/
3 dysthymic disorder/
4 or/1–3
5 exp antidepressive agents/
6 antidepressant$.tw.
7 or/5–6
8 4 and 7

In journal articles it may not be possible to describe the search in great detail, but a thesis or report should have the space to include all the search strategies in an appendix. In a journal article it is always possible, even if the description of the search has to be brief, to indicate that full search details are available from the author.

CONCLUSIONS

Literature reviews place new research within the context of existing research. A comprehensive literature search informing a review ensures that, as far as possible, new research does not duplicate, unwittingly, past efforts. A systematic review based on a thorough literature search can show where new research is needed and where uncertainty about clinical effectiveness remains. Given the importance of the literature search for the review, it is essential to record its conduct in as much detail as the final publication allows. The quality of the literature search in the production of literature reviews and in identifying the need for primary research, is becoming a key area of focus for readers and peer reviewers as they assess the overall quality of published research. Researchers can make sure that the effort invested in this part of the research is reflected by a clear and explicit account of the search methods.

KEY POINTS

Carrying out a systematic review is a major undertaking. It involves:

- Defining a clear research question and criteria for inclusion/selection of studies.
- Identifying the databases and other sources to be searched.
- Preparing comprehensive search strategies.
- Recording the progress of the searches conducted.
- Documenting the searches.
- Disseminating the findings.

REFERENCES

1. Mulrow, C. Rationale for systematic reviews. In: *Systematic reviews* (Chalmers, I., Altman, D.H. eds.), 1995; pp. 1–8. British Medical Journal Publishing, London.
2. Cook, D. J., Mulrow, C. D., Haynes, R. B. Systematic reviews: synthesis of best evidence for clinical decisions. *Annals of Internal Medicine*, 1997; **126,** 376–80.
3. NHS Centre for Reviews and Dissemination *Undertaking systematic reviews of research on effectiveness. CRD Guidelines for those carrying out or commissioning reviews.* 1996; NHS Centre for Reviews and Dissemination.
4. Goodman, C. *Literature searching and evidence interpretation for assessing health care practices.* 1993; Swedish Council on Technology Assessment in Health care. Also available full text at: http://www.sbu.se/sbu-site/reports/alphabetical.html

5. The Cochrane Collaboration The Cochrane Handbook. In: *The Cochrane Library* [database on disk and CDROM]. 1996; Update Software. Updated quarterly.
6. Huang, M. P., Alessi, N. *Psychiatry navigates the Web*. 1995; Available at: http://www.psych.med.umich.edu/web/psytimes/psychwww.htm
7. Greenhalgh, T. How to read a paper: the MEDLINE database. *British Medical Journal*. 1997; **315**, 180–3.
8. Dickersin, K., Scherer, R., Lefebvre. C. Identifying relevant studies for systematic reviews. In: *Systematic reviews* (Chalmer, I., Altman, D. H. eds.), 1995; pp. 17–36, BMJ Publishing, London.
9. Crombie, I. K. *The pocket guide to critical appraisal*. 1996; BMJ Publishing, London.

Chapter Five

Writing a research protocol

Stephen Curran

INTRODUCTION

Writing a protocol is an important part of the research process which is easy to overlook and tempting to avoid. It is sometimes difficult to put your ideas down on paper and it is common to feel anxious about having these ideas 'criticized'. A good protocol will take some time to prepare but it will ultimately facilitate the smooth running of your research. Why then should you take the trouble to write a protocol rather than 'getting on' with the research? The main purpose of a protocol is to help you to be clear about the general aims of your study and the specific hypotheses you wish to test. Writing a protocol is a key element in this and this chapter will illustrate how to complete a protocol and use it successfully to take your research forward. There can be several benefits associated with writing a protocol. It is harder to avoid important issues when something has to be written down (e.g. what is my hypothesis?). It will force you to think through the various aspects of your study including the title, your aims and hypothesis and the methodology. It also has the benefit of helping you identify problems before they arise and increases the likelihood that the study will be successfully completed and published. The protocol can also form the basis of an Ethics Committee proposal, a submission to a university department for a postgraduate degree or a grant proposal.

For all these reasons writing a protocol is considered to be an important exercise by experienced researchers.[1] More detailed discussions of protocol preparation have been published.[2–8] In summary, it:

- Makes your ideas explicit.
- Enables others to read/comment on your ideas.
- Facilitates the exchange of ideas.
- Helps identify potential problems early on.
- May form the basis of other proposals (e.g. an ethics committee submission and provide a basic structure for summarizing your work for publication).

GETTING STARTED – IDENTIFYING THE RESEARCH QUESTION

Some topics, such as psychotherapy, are intrinsically more difficult to research. Whatever the area of research, one of the keys to successful research is to keep your ideas simple; however, formulating a suitable question can sometimes be difficult. As Goldberg has noted[9]

> 'it is relatively easy to think of questions to which no-one knows the answer; the trick is to think of one that could be illuminated by a single person working in their spare time which hasn't already been answered'.

It is also highly likely that you will have very limited or non-existent resources. How can the specific question be formulated and assessed using the time and resources available to you?

In order to begin to generate ideas for research, some find it useful to keep a small note book handy to record potential research ideas as they come to you. These ideas may be strengthened after reading journal articles or after other meetings such as journal clubs or case conferences. Talking about and discussing your ideas with friends, colleagues and more senior members of staff can help to consolidate your research idea. The College reading list is a very good source of preliminary information and The College Library staff can also help by undertaking small literature reviews.

Try to focus on a project that will be relatively easy to conduct. This will be more successful if it can be incorporated into your routine clinical work. It will also be easier if the topic under consideration is relatively common (e.g. most will find it easier to access patients with depression than to try to recruit a sample of patients with Creutzfeld Jakob disease).

One difficulty is that you need to answer a specific question, however, it is commonly the case that you will initially have insufficient knowledge about the area to formulate this question. One way you could approach this problem would be to do it in stages using the 'Funnel approach' (Figure 5.1). Ask yourself:

- Which area would you like to do research in (e.g. child and adolescent, old age, or general psychiatry?). This is usually straightforward as you will probably want to do your research in the area in which you eventually want to specialize. Let's assume you choose old age psychiatry.
- You might then consider the broad theme you would like to concentrate on (e.g. epidemiology, clinical features, assessment, diagnosis, aetiology, treatment or prognosis). This decision might take a little longer. If there is someone locally in one of these areas you could discuss this with him or her.
- If you choose to do your research on 'treatment' you would then need to decide on which sort of treatment. This would be either a psychological or physical treatment. Further discussions with colleagues and a

potential supervisor might lead you to opt for physical treatments. Then you would need to narrow the area down further. For example:

- Choose from drugs, electroconvulsive therapy or psychosurgery. Some general reading and further discussions will help you to choose one of these three main areas of physical treatment. Clearly, work involving psychosurgery would be more difficult to organize for most trainees than one involving a small project dealing with some aspect of the use of neuroleptics or the logistical aspects of monitoring side-effects.
- If you decided to examine the 'drug' option, which drug or group of drugs would you like to investigate and which aspect (e.g. compliance, side-effects, efficacy etc.) would you like to study? Again, further reading and discussion will help you to focus on something more specific. General textbooks on drug treatments in psychiatry including the different classes of drugs, mechanisms of actions and side-effects will give you a broad overview. Keep copies of everything you read as these will be useful for subsequent publications/theses.
- You might decide that lithium appears to be an interesting 'drug' and one which has been poorly studied compared with many other psychoactive drugs. At this stage it would be appropriate to do some general reading focused on lithium including identifying and reading specific articles. Review articles are particularly helpful in this respect. Your reading around the subject would help to clarify your thoughts.
- You might decide that it would be interesting to examine an aspect of the side-effects of lithium. After further reading, thought and discussion (preferably with your supervisor at this stage) the general aim of your study might be *to investigate the relationship between side-effects of lithium and lithium plasma levels*. This will give you a firm sense of what you wish to investigate and this aim (which by definition is still quite broad in nature) can be discussed further with your supervisor.
- After additional reading (which should be focused) you will be able to develop your hypothesis. Your hypothesis might be *there is no association between the side-effects of lithium and lithium plasma levels at 12 hours post-dose.*

This 'funnel approach' (Figure 5.1) where a broad area is gradually focused down into a specific research question is only one way that you might arrive at a hypothesis to investigate. One reason why trainees have difficulty developing hypotheses that can be realistically be tested is that the process is quite complex. Working through the funnel approach to form a specific hypothesis will require much thought, time, reading and discussion. Generally speaking it is unusual for most people doing research for the first time to be able to formulate a hypothesis 'out of thin air', but the step-by step process outlined above may help you achieve this.

Figure 5.1 *An example of the 'Funnel approach' when choosing a research question: this starts with a broad area (old age psychiatry) and eventually focuses on a specific hypothesis.*

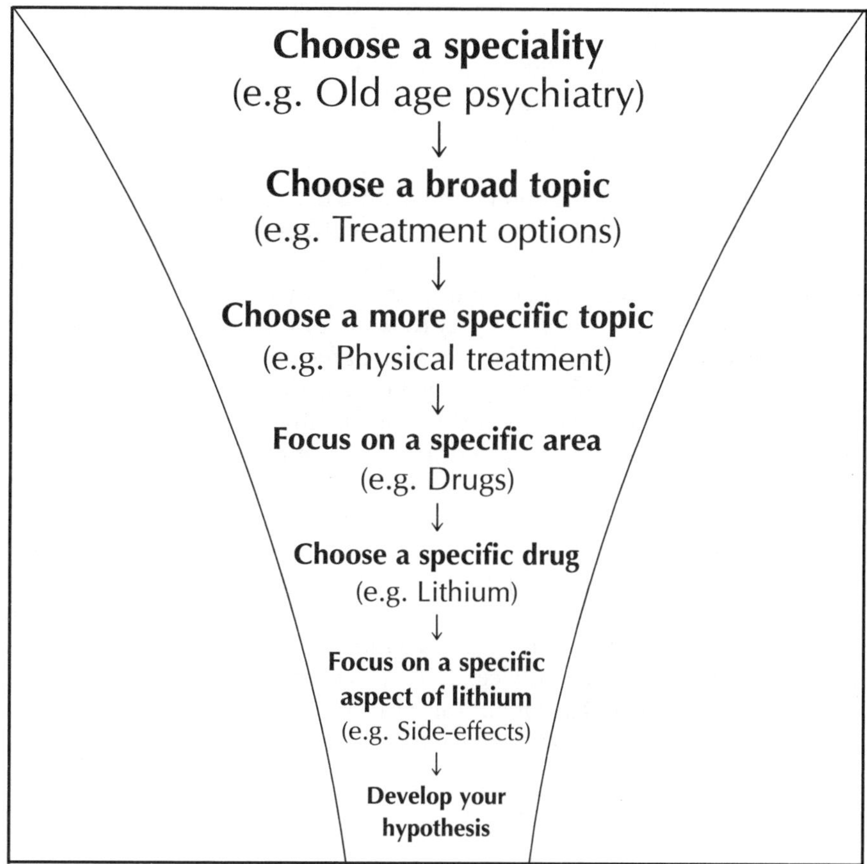

Formulating the research question does take time, but this is time well spent. This process also emphasizes the need for reading around the subject which gradually results in the research question becoming focused. It also emphasizes the need for discussion with colleagues. Despite this, at this stage you should still consider both your aims and hypotheses as 'drafts'. Once you have had a chance to write the methodology section, together with further discussions and reading, you might feel that your original hypothesis was still unclear or too ambitious. If so, amend it in the light of this.

Now you can start writing your protocol. This should be no longer than two to three sides of A4 (usually single space) unless you have been asked to write more (e.g. for a grant proposal).

WRITING THE PROTOCOL

The principal elements of a protocol are summarized in Table 5.1. Writing a protocol can be quite difficult to get started. It is helpful to start by making a note of the main headings as outlined in Table 5.1 as this will give the protocol (or research proposal) some structure. The first draft can be the most difficult and the first two or three drafts are often best written in 'privacy'. Don't worry too much about how 'awful' the first draft appears to be. Once something is on paper you will find it easier to make corrections and by rewording the protocol it will help you to clarify your thoughts. Very quickly it will begin to look more like a formal protocol. Don't expect to produce an excellent protocol after a couple of hours. This is a very important part of the research process and needs time to do it well. Expect to write/discuss and re-write/further discuss the protocol several times before agreeing a final version. There may be a desire to avoid re-writing the protocol and 'get on with the study', however, time invested at this stage is time very well spent. Many people find it helpful to put each draft to one side for a day or so before re-reading and re-writing it. Ask others to read your protocol for an independent assessment after you have revised it several times (e.g. a partner, close colleague, a consultant you are working with or a local academic with an interest in the field). Although you may be anxious about being criticized, constructive criticism is preferable at this stage rather than after the study has been completed. Trainees often complain that they get conflicting advice. If this occurs, discuss the conflicting advice with those who gave it and/or with somebody neutral. If necessary bring the two conflicting colleagues together.

Table 5.1 *Key features of a research protocol*

- Title.
- List of investigators/collaborators.
- Brief introduction:
    - Brief outline of previous research.
    - Why does this study need to be done?
    - How does it differ from previous work?
- Aims and hypotheses.
- Methodology:
    - Study design.
    - Patients (e.g. recruitment, assessment).
    - Materials/rating scales etc. used.
    - Statistical procedures.
    - Logistics (e.g. costs, time to complete).
- Ethics Committee/ethical issues.
- Dissemination (e.g. publication, conference, presentations (etc).

THE DETAILED CONTENT OF THE PROTOCOL

1. Title

This should reflect the general aim and specific hypothesis of the study and should enable others to get a feel for your study by simply reading the title. In general you should avoid abbreviations and it should not be too long (maximum 12–15 words). For example, you are likely to be no clearer about a study entitled, *Non-monotonic effects of test illuminance on CFFT; a study of Fo. light adaptation with annular surrounds.* However, one entitled, *A comparison of clock and pentagon drawing in Alzheimer's disease* would be much clearer. It is highly likely that the title will be revised or changed by the time the protocol has been completed.

2. Investigators/collaborators

This is an important but often neglected aspect of the protocol. It indicates who will be involved with the study and also suggests who will be on the final publication. It is better to clarify these issues at this time rather than later when arguments can occur, particularly when multiple authors are involved. Your supervisor would traditionally be last on the protocol (and paper) and the individual doing the bulk of the work (study design, data collection and analysis and writing) would be first author. In the methodology section you can clarify (very briefly) what each collaborator will be doing. There are a number of advantages to collaborating with several colleagues. First, you will get peer group support from your colleagues and secondly, you can divide the work up enabling you either to complete the study sooner or complete a larger study in the same time.

3. Introduction/background

A very brief introduction which sets the scene for your research idea is very helpful, particularly for those who will be asked to comment on your protocol. It should not be a detailed review of the literature (this would come later either in your thesis or subsequent publication). It should succinctly summarize the literature you have read and will logically provide the background leading to your aims and hypotheses. It is useful to include a comment about why this particular study needs to be done and how it differs from previous studies. You are unlikely to get to this position without a detailed review of the literature, but only a brief synopsis needs to be included in your protocol. If this is subsequently written-up as a thesis the introduction might be 25–50 pages long, but an important aspect of the protocol is brevity and this should be reflected in the introduction.

4. Aims and hypotheses

The aim of the study is a general statement about what you intend to do (e.g. examine the relationship between serum lithium levels and side-effects). It will help to orientate the reader to the focus of your study. Hypotheses, on the other hand, are very much more specific (e.g. *'there is no association between serum lithium levels one hour after taking lithium and hand tremor')*. For any given study, the number of hypotheses should be kept to a minimum. It is also important that your hypotheses are clearly stated in *advance* of the research. As Hirsch (1992) has noted,[10] 'discoveries made in the course of the research or at the time of the analysis of the results are not true results in the sense that they do not test hypotheses which have been formulated before.'

5. Methods

This is perhaps the most important part of the protocol and should make up the largest part. The principal 'test' for the methodology section is whether the methods you have chosen enable you to test the hypothesis (es) that have been established in advance.[10] If you are planning to undertake a clinical study and will be using rating or measuring instruments you could divide this section into Patients and Materials. There are a number of questions that you should address, but this is by no means an exhaustive list:

- What experimental design will be used (see Chapter 3).
- Where will the patients come from (e.g. community based, inpatients)?
- What sampling procedures will you use?
- How representative will your patients be (e.g. of a particular condition)?
- What numbers will you need?
- How will patients be identified (e.g. diagnostic criteria)?
- Will there be any inclusion or exclusion criteria?
- Where will patients be assessed and by whom?
- How long will the assessment take?
- Does the investigator need any special training?

You must describe the questionnaires and rating scales or other means of measurement and state why these have been selected. Are these measures *valid* and *reliable* for your purposes? The validity of a test concerns what the test measures and how well it does so. Reliability refers to the consistency of scores obtained when the same sample is tested again using the same test on different occasions (test–re-test reliability), or by a different rater (inter-rater reliability). Other measures of reliability include the comparison of different sets of equivalent items, and examining the impact of using the same test under variable examining conditions.

If you are using a measure you have developed or are using an established measure in a different context you will need to show that the instrument is valid and reliable in the group you are proposing to investigate. This might be a study in its own right!

Other practical issues concerning your research that must be addressed include:

- Is the proposal a pilot or main study?
- How will terms be defined? Definitions need to be explicitly stated and not left to the readers imagination. What is meant by 'depression', 'anxiety' or 'panic attacks'? What is meant by 'patients will have a full assessment' or be 'carefully evaluated'.

At the end of this section, anyone wishing to repeat your methodology should be able to do so, since repetition of studies is part of the normal process of research. Findings of major significance are usually repeated several times, by independent investigators, before a novel finding becomes accepted. For this reason definitions and descriptions need to be clear (or appropriately referenced, e.g. DSM-IV criteria for major depression). An example of a protocol is included in Table 5.2. This is still at a 'draft' stage. Try to identify 'good' and 'poor' aspects of the protocol. Some suggestions discussing its strengths and weaknesses are found at the end of the protocol.

Table 5.2 *Draft protocol and comments to improve its content and structure*

The ability of CFFT, a neuropsychophysical method based on the continuous method of limits, to distinguish between community based patients living in their own homes over the age of 65 with mild-moderate AD and MID based on the DSM-IV diagnostic criteria.

Background

SDAT is a common and devastating illness that initially deprives the person of recent memory and causes enormous stress and suffering for patients and their families. It results in total dependence on other people and patients eventually die. In AD, extensive and irreversible brain damage generally occurs before clinical symptoms become apparent. In order to obtain maximum benefit from currently available treatments for AD, it is essential to be able to ascertain which people have pre-clinical AD before there is widespread cortical atrophy. The availability of drugs for the treatment of AD has made the need for *early detection* of crucial importance. If drugs are given early in the course of the disease there would be more hope of arresting or significantly slowing the progress of the condition and this would be of immense benefit to patients, their relatives and to society. Giving such a drug at a later stage would probably be ineffective and at best would prolong disability, and might increase the personal and financial costs of AD. There is therefore a pressing need for non-invasive, easy to use and inexpensive means of *screening* people at risk of developing AD. There are a variety of possible ways of detecting early AD including neuroimaging techniques, but these tend to be very cumbersome, expensive or invasive and potentially dangerous (e.g. lumbar pucture). In addition, these techniques are only available in a few research centres and not to community-based healthy subjects. ▶

CFFT is a well established neurophysiological technique that has been shown to reflect brain cortical activity. In neuropsychological terms it is regarded as a measure of the information processing capacity of the central nervous system (CNS) and has been extensively investigated in both young and elderly healthy subjects. The authors have examined this measure in a number of previous studies. The test has also been shown to be a *valid* and *reliable* measure of CNS function in patients with AD. It is also *quick* and *easy to administer* and is relatively *inexpensive.* It can be used easily in *community*-based settings (e.g. patients' homes, GP practices) and is very *portable* (size of a small brief case). It also requires *minimal training,* has no *floor* or *ceiling* effects and it is not influenced by *cultural* or *educational* factors (it is a psychophysical threshold). In addition, it provides an *objective* and *quantitative* measure of CNS function. It is also free of many of the methodological problems associated with rating scales.

Purpose

The authors believe that CFFT would be helpful in identifying early cases of AD, i.e. before clinical symptoms became apparent. To test this hypothesis would involve screening a large sample (approximately 1500) of healthy elderly subjects and then reassess them at regular intervals over several years. This would be a large and expensive study and further work on CFFT needs to be undertaken before commencing a study of this size. CFFT satisfies many of the requirements needed in a test which would be used for this purpose (see above). In addition, it is not sensitive to increasing age in elderly subjects (Curran *et al.,* 1990). If CFFT was affected by both AD and increasing age it would then be difficult to interpret CFFT data in patients developing AD, i.e. very early cases. This is important as early dementia is often indistinguishable from normal ageing. However, since there are now drugs available for the treatment of AD (but not MID, the other principal cause of dementia) it would be important for such a test to be able to distinguish between AD and MID (one would not wish to commence a drug in patients with MID as there would be no clinical benefit and patients might be at increased risk from side-effects). Thus, the purpose of the present study is to determine whether CFFT is able to distinguish between patients with mild-moderate AD and MID.

Plan of research work

We would plan to assess 40 patients with AD or MID (20 of each) and examine the behaviour of CFFT in these two conditions. Patients will be assessed from a variety of settings, e.g. patients' homes, outpatient clinic, day hospital and dementia assessment wards. The *clinical assessment* will involve taking a medical and psychiatric history, a physical examination, laboratory investigations (a routine dementia blood screen) and a CT scan. Diagnosis will be based on DSM-IV diagnostic criteria (APA, 1994). Only patients with mild-moderate AD or MID will be included. CT scans would normally only be undertaken on a small proportion of patients (as part of the routine diagnostic work-up in dementia) but for diagnostic rigor, a CT scan will need to be performed on all patients included in the study. Patients with AD and MID will be matched for age, gender and degree of cognitive impairment as determined by the Mini-Mental State Examination (Folstein *et al.,* 1975). Patients who successfully ▶

complete this part of the assessment will then be assessed using CFFT and several neuropsychological tests on a subsequent occasion so as not to over burden the patient. To measure CFFT, the patient will be asked to sit in front of a small console (the size of a brief case) and asked to look at four small red lights (1 cm square). Patients will be required to press a button when they perceive that the lights have either started or stopped flickering. Several well established *neuropsychological* measures will also be administered which have been demonstrated to reflect specific cortical lobe function known to be impaired in patients with AD. The administration of CFFT and the neuropsychological tests will take approximately 45 minutes. Protocols are available for all these measures to ensure standardized administration. Before formally testing subjects, the purpose of the study will be explained to patients and their consent will be obtained. Consent from the patient's next of kin (NOK) and GP will also be obtained. An information sheet will be available for the patient and the patient's NOK and GP. The ability of all these measures to distinguish between AD and MID will be determined using SPSS version 6.1.

References

American Psychiatric Association (1994) Diagnostic and Statistical Manual of Mental Disorders, Fourth Edition, Washington, D.C.

Curran, S., Wattis, J.P., Shillingford, C. and Hindmarch, I. (1990). Critical flicker fusion in normal elderly subjects; a cross-sectional community study (I). Current Psychology: Research and Reviews, 9, 1, 25–34.

Folstein, M.F., Folstein, S.E. and McHugh, P.R. (1975) 'Mini-mental State'. A practical method for grading the cognitive state of patients for the clinician. Journal of Psychiatric Research, 12, 189–198.

Lezak, M.D. (1983) Neuropsychological Assessment (Second Edition), New York, Oxford University Press.

Comments on the draft protocol

This protocol is at an early draft stage and requires further revision.

- The title is too long and is not very clear. Avoid abbreviations in titles.
- The investigator(s) needs to be included with his/her job title and professional address.
- Abbreviations, when used for the first time, should be spelt out in full.
- It is not clear what CFFT is and what it measures.
- There are no aims or hypotheses.
- The study design is not clear.
- Will the proposed number of patients give the study sufficient power?
- No mention is made about sampling procedures.
- Will this be a representative sample of patients with Alzheimer's disease and Multi-infarct dementia?
- The protocol should include clear inclusion or exclusion criteria.
- How long will all the assessments take and who will do them?
- Will the assessments be done at the same time? and in the same order (order effects)? ▶

- Details about the neuropsychological tests should be given (e.g. which ones will be used, are they suitable for this purpose and are they valid and reliable?).
- Details should be given about the data analysis (e.g. ANOVA) rather than which statistical package will be used (this is irrelevant).
- Details about Ethics Committee submission are needed.
- Further details about resources, costs and logistics are needed to demonstrate that these important areas have been considered.
- The literature review could be strengthened by adding further references, particularly about CFFT.

---

6. Statistics

Planning the analysis of the study is also an important part of the methodology and should not be left until after the study has been completed. You should address:

- How will the data be collected and what sort of data will they be (e.g. ordinal data such as mood rating scales) or interval data (e.g. temperature using the centigrade scale)?
- What numbers or sample size will you need?
- How do you propose to analyse the data?

Except for very simple studies, it is important to seek the advice of a statistician. Although this can be very frustrating if you are told that your proposal will have insufficient numbers to demonstrate a significant result, it is infinitely better to be told this at the protocol writing stage than after the study has been completed. The basics of statistical analysis are summarized in Chapters 6, 7 and 8.

7. Logistics, resources and costs

This is an important component of the protocol. For the study to be successful you need to think through the potential resource/logistic implications including:

- How much time do you have available to undertake the research?
- How many patients do you intend to include in the study?
- Can this number be recruited in the time available to complete the study?
- How long will it take to assess patients?
- Will there be any cost/resource implications?

Try to suggest a start and finishing date for your proposal. Writing down a clear timetable can be a useful method to help you plan and check your progress. The cost or resource implications of your study may be very small, but you may still need to undertake a large amount of photocopying. If this is the case you might simply need to obtain permission to do your photocopying in your own department, but you should at least give this some thought before you start collecting data. It is also helpful to keep a research file on each patient/subject you include in your study in order to record your information. This information should be regarded as confidential and kept in a secure place. Make sure that the information is well organized since if you return to this file some time later you may have difficulty understanding what you did!

8. Ethics committee

Generally speaking, studies involving patients and particularly those in which procedures are undertaken (e.g. rating scale) which are not part of the normal clinical process should be submitted to the Ethics Committee. If in doubt submit. It is often possible to speak to the chairman of the Ethics Committee (or his or her representative) to get advice on this process. You could let him or her have a copy of your proposal and ask whether a formal submission to the committee is necessary. It is important to note that if ethics committee approval is necessary, this might delay your study by several months. Several Trusts also now have a Research Directorate and this body might wish to approve *all* studies undertaken on patients within your Trusts (see Chapter 12 for more details about ethical aspects of study design and Ethics Committees).

Once you have written the protocol, discussed it with colleagues and your supervisor and revised it several times you may find that the protocol looks very different from your original draft. You will now be in a much better position to carry out your research idea with success. The time you have invested in writing your protocol will mean that your study is more likely to run smoothly and you are more likely to get it published.

KEY POINTS

- This is a vital component of the research process and will help you to decide what you want to do and how you will do it.
- Allocate sufficient time.
- Choose the research question to be answered carefully.
- Seek constructive comments from your colleagues (it is better to have your study 'criticized' at this stage rather than after the study has been completed).
- Discuss your protocol with your supervisor.
- The protocol will probably have to be re-written several times.
- Use the process of writing a protocol to clarify and improve your study.

REFERENCES

1. Freeman, C., Tyrer, P. Getting started in research. In: *Research Methods in Psychiatry; A Beginner's Guide,* 2nd edn, (Freeman, C., Tyrer, P., eds), 1992; pp 1–11. Gaskell, London.
2. Kane, E. *Doing Your Own Research; Basic Descriptive Research in the Social Sciences and Humanities.* 1993; Marion Boyars, London.
3. O' Connor, M., Woodford, F. P. *Writing Scientific Papers in English.* 1977; Pitman Medical, London.
4. Paton, A. Write a paper. In: *How to do it, Volume 2.* 1985; pp. 207–11. British Medical Journal, London.
5. Stephen, J. Search the literature. In: *How to do it, Volume 3.* 1985; pp. 77–82. British Medical Journal, London.
6. Stephen, J. Carry out an on line search. In: *How to do it, Volume 3.* 1985; pp. 83–88. British Medical Journal, London.
7. Warren, M. D. Plan a research project. In: *How to do it, Volume 2.* 1985; pp. 117–21. British Medical Journal, London.
8. Johns, L. Use a word processor. In: *How to do it, Volume 3.* 1985; pp. 89–93. British Medical Journal, London.
9. Goldberg, D. Planning psychiatric research. In: *A Handbook for Trainee Psychiatrists.* (Rix, K. J. B. ed.), 1987; pp. 256–69. Bailliere Tindall, London.
10. Hirsch, S. R. The rationale of clinical trials. In: *The Scientific Basis of Psychiatry,* 2nd edn. (Weller, M. P .I., Eysenck, M. W., eds), pp. 65–74. 1992; W. B. Saunders Co Ltd, London.

Chapter Six

Descriptive statistics

Tom Hughes

INTRODUCTION

The statistics in this chapter are straightforward and will allow you to summarize and describe your key results. It is not necessary to be a mathematical expert to understand basic statistics even if you have not previously used statistics.

DESCRIPTIVE AND INFERENTIAL STATISTICS

When you have completed your fieldwork, you will have gathered a set of data, usually in the form of figures. In research, data are recorded on a *sample* of subjects taken from a *target population* and related to a *reference population*. This chapter will help you to describe your sample.

It is useful to be able to describe the data from your sample in a brief and accurate way without having to read them all out. *Descriptive statistics* are those used in describing sets of data and are the subject of this chapter. The chapter will cover:

- Different kinds of data.
- Measures of average.
- Measures of the variation of scores in a data set.
- The distribution of the data.
- The normal distribution.
- Skew.
- The special property of the *standard deviation* of a normal distribution.

Inferential statistics are concerned with drawing conclusions from your data and are not dealt with here. They are summarized in detail in Chapters 7 and 8.

THE DIFFERENT KINDS OF DATA

1. Categorical or nominal data

These are data where each observation is allocated to one of two or more 'named' categories, e.g.

- Male/female.
- Depressed/not depressed.
- Pregnant/not pregnant.
- House numbers in a street.
- The numbers on the shirts of players in a football team (from 1 to 11).

Data in different categories are *qualitatively*, but not quantitatively, different from each other (see Chapter 3). Nominal data can be in numerical form as in the last two examples above, or converted to numerical form using a code (e.g. score male as 0 and female as 1).

2. Continuous data

Different scores from a continuous data set are *quantitatively* different from each other. There are three kinds of continuous data:

- Ordinal data are those where a difference in score indicates a difference in order or rank (e.g. first, second and third in a race). The difference between each score is not necessarily the same (e.g. the difference in race time between first and second is not necessarily equal to that between second and third).
- Interval data are also those where a difference in score indicates a difference in order or rank, but also the difference between any two adjacent scores on an interval scale is always the same (i.e. the difference between 1 and 2 is the same as between 2 and 3, e.g. the Celsius scale of temperature).
- Ratio data are almost the same as interval data, with the exception that on a ratio scale there is an absolute zero (e.g. the Kelvin scale of temperature, or the time after an event).

PROPERTIES OF DIFFERENT KINDS OF DATA

Neither nominal data in numerical form nor ordinal data can be added or subtracted, multiplied or divided (or you could do so, but the number you obtained would be meaningless). Interval and ratio data can be added, subtracted, multiplied or divided.

DISTRIBUTION

A distribution is a collection of scores (e.g. intelligence quotient (IQ) scores in a group of subjects). Implicit in the term distribution is that some scores occur more frequently in your data than others. A *frequency distribution* is a collection of scores plotted in graphical form so that the number of times each score occurs is shown (Figure 6.1). The data in Figure 6.1 are in the form of a *histogram*. An alternative way of plotting the graph would be to plot the mid-point of each of the bars in the form of a line.

Figure 6.1 *Distribution of IQ scores*

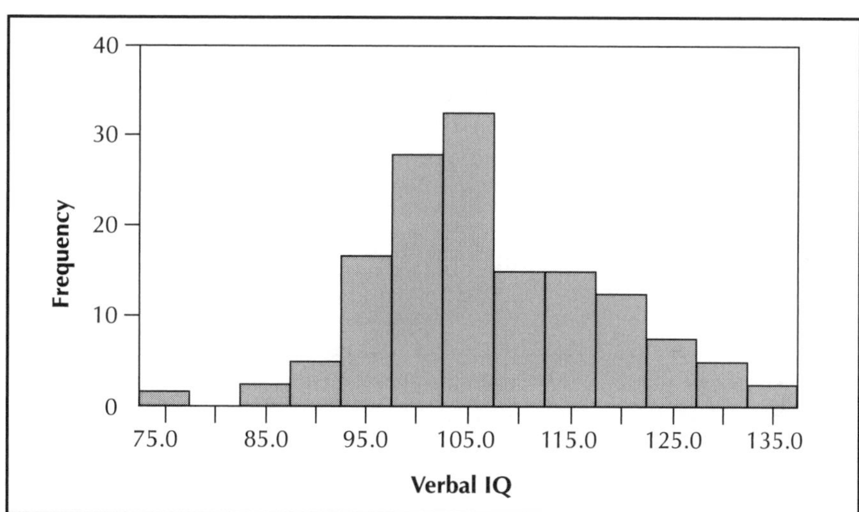

THE NORMAL DISTRIBUTION

This is an important concept in statistics. The normal distribution is also referred to as the *Gaussian distribution*, after a mathematician. A normal distribution is shown as a histogram in Figure 6.1. The normal distribution has a number of properties. It is:

- Bell-shaped.
- Symmetrical about the mean (i.e. if you drew a line down the centre of the distribution, each side forms a mirror image of the other).
- The mean, median and mode are equal (see below for definition of these terms).
- The 'tails' of the curve theoretically never touch the horizontal axis of the graph, and continue to infinity.

MEASURES OF AVERAGE OR 'CENTRAL TENDENCY'

You will probably be used to using a 'measure of central tendency' to describe data and these are often referred to as an *average*. There are three kinds of average, the *mean*, the *median*, and the *mode*, which you can use to describe the data in your distribution.

- The mean is the sum of the values of the individual scores, divided by the total number of scores or Σ (X_1, X_2, X_3 etc.) $\div$ n, where Σ means 'the sum of', X is each score and n is the total number of scores. Thus the mean of the scores 5, 7, 8, 11, 11, 13 and 15 is 10.
- The median is the middle value of the scores when the scores are placed in rank order of magnitude (i.e. in rank order from the lowest to the highest score). If there is an even number of scores, there may be two middle values, in which case the median is the average (i.e. the mean) of those two values. In the above example, the median score is 11.
- The mode is the score which occurs most frequently. There can be more than one mode. In the above example, the mode is 11.

You should use the average which most accurately describes your data. The mean is most often used. However, if your data are *skewed* (see below), the median is generally a better description.

Example:

A way of seeing something similar to the effect of skewing data is to consider the following data set:

1, 2, 3, 4, 5, 6, 7

Here, the number of scores (n) = 7. The mean and the median are both 4. If the number 7 was changed to 100, the mean would change dramatically, but the median would remain unaltered.

If your data are ordinal data, you should use the median, because to find the mean would involve addition and division of the scores, which you cannot do with ordinal data.

The mode is less often used but can be useful, particularly in addition to one of the other measures, and if there is more than one mode.

MEASURES OF SPREAD

In addition to describing the average of your data, it is useful to have a measure of how spread out your scores are. These are the *range* and the *standard deviation*. The *range* is the difference between the top score and the bottom score (e.g. a range of 6 in the last example). This is frequently used, together with the median, in describing skewed data. Alternatively, the *interquartile range* can be used. This is the difference between the 25th and 75th centile scores, and is more useful than the range if the top or bottom scores are *outliers* (i.e. very different from the other scores). To calculate this, you must first work out the *lower and upper quartiles*:

The *lower quartile* is the (N+1/4)th result when they are arranged in order. In this example, this is the second result in rank order = 2.

The *upper quartile* is the ((N+1) × 3/4)th result when they are arranged in order. In this example, this is the sixth result in rank order = 6. Thus the *inter-quartile range* is 6–2 = 4.

Before considering the standard deviation, let us consider something called the *mean deviation* (or average difference). The mean deviation is the *average (mean) difference of each score from the mean* (i.e. the sum of the individual differences of each score from the mean, divided by the total number of scores), or:

$$\text{The mean deviation} = \Sigma\ [(\underline{X}-X) \div n]$$

Some of the scores will be greater than the mean, and some less than the mean. So, some of these differences will be negative, and some positive. In a normal distribution there are the same number of scores above and below the mean, and the positive differences equal the negative differences. The mean deviation is then zero, which does not tell you much about the spread of your scores. In order to convey some useful information about your data, you will want to get rid of the effect of the positive and negative signs. Multiplying two negative numbers together results in a positive number. If we square all the differences from the mean (i.e. multiply each difference by itself), all the negative differences will become positive differences. If we then add all these differences (which gives the *sum of the squares*) and divide by the total number of scores ,we have the *mean of the sum of the squares* (also called the *variance*).

$$\text{The variance} = (\Sigma\ (\underline{X}-X)^2 \div n)$$

Because we squared all the differences, the figure we now have must be 'unsquared', i.e. we take the square root of the variance to obtain the *standard deviation*. In mathematical terms, this can be written as:

$$\text{The standard deviation} = \sqrt{}(\Sigma\ (\underline{X}-X)^2 \div n)$$

where √ = square root
Σ = 'the sum of '
$\underline{X}$ = the population mean score
X = each individual score
n = the number of subjects in the population

So, the standard deviation is just the average (mean) difference of the scores from the average (mean), with a bit of statistical jiggery-pokery to remove the negative signs. The standard deviation has units. For example, if you are measuring age, the mean age of your sample may be 40 years, and one standard deviation may be 5 years.

Of course, you will never have to calculate the SD (or in fact most statistics) yourself. A calculator or computer will do this for you. What you do need to do is seek to *understand* the relevance of any results.

A small complication with the standard deviation

In most research, you work with a sample of the population, so that there will be a degree of inaccuracy in your value for the standard deviation of your sample when used to estimate the standard deviation in the target population. This is taken into account by making the standard deviation a little larger, as shown in the formula below:

For a sample, the standard deviation = $\sqrt{(\Sigma\,(\underline{X}-X)^2 \div (n-1)\,)}$

DEVIATIONS FROM 'NORMAL': SKEW, KURTOSIS, MORE THAN ONE MODE

Your data may not have a 'normal distribution' because there are a lot of low scores, or a lot of high scores. In this case, your data is said to be *skewed*. Figure 6.2 shows data which is *positively* skewed, and Figure 6.3 data which is *negatively* skewed.

Figure 6.2 *Positively skewed data*

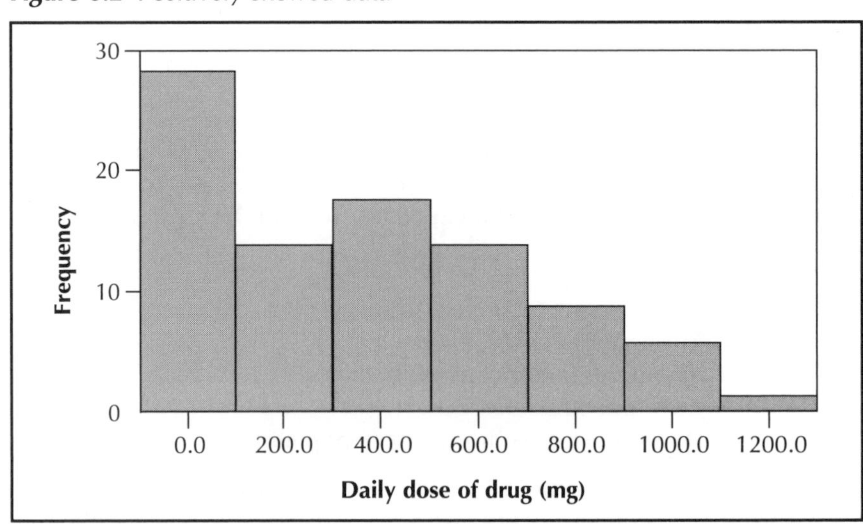

Figure 6.3 *Negatively skewed data*

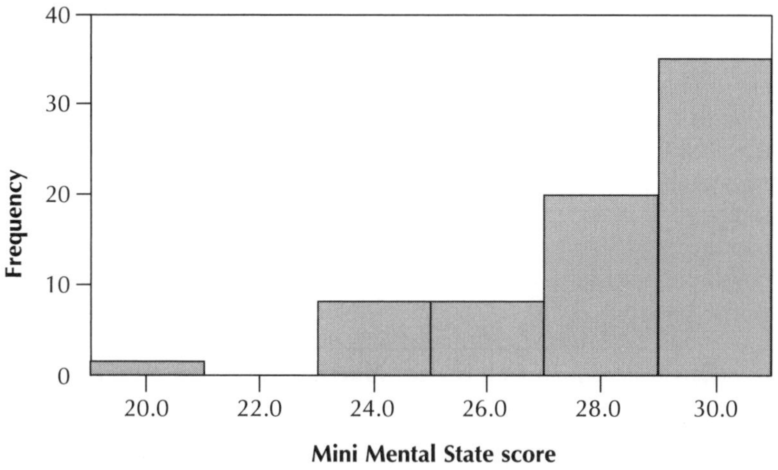

To remember which is which:

- In negatively skewed data, the first part of the slope is horizontal like the minus sign –.
- In positively skewed data the first part of the slope is vertical, like the vertical line on the plus sign +.

In addition:

- The curve may be flattened on the top (*platykuric*).
- The curve may be more pointed than the normal curve (*leptokuric*).
- A curve with one 'peak' such as occurs in the normal distribution is *unimodal*, but the curve may be *bimodal* etc.

The names of the types of distribution are not important, but:

- You need to know what the shape of the distribution is to decide how to describe it (e.g. whether to use the mean or median).
- You need to know whether your data are normal or not before you decide which statistical tests to use to analyse it. The easiest way to tell whether your data are normal or not is to plot it out in a graph and this can easily be achieved by using a computer and looking at its distribution on the screen.

ARE MY DATA 'NORMAL'?

When you look at the distribution of a variable from your data on the computer screen, it probably won't look quite like the 'normal' distribution.

- It does not really matter whether the variable in your sample forms a normal distribution or not. What matters is whether your sample *comes from a target population* where that variable is normally distributed.
- A variable which is normally distributed in the target population may not be exactly normally distributed in your sample, because of *random variation* in your sample. In other words, if you took a lot of samples of water from a pond, the contents of each sample would vary a little from each other.
- You have to make a judgement about whether it is reasonable to assume that the data are normally distributed in the target population, from looking at the shape of the distribution in your sample, and this is not an exact science. Your computer software will usually be able to provide figures based on statistical tests which will estimate what the chances are that the variable is normally distributed in the target population.

THE NORMAL DISTRIBUTION AND THE STANDARD DEVIATION

For data which are normally distributed, but not other data, the standard deviation can convey some extra, very useful, information. Roughly two-thirds (actually 68.2%) of all scores lie within one standard deviation on either side of the mean score, and roughly 95% of scores lie within 2 standard deviations on either side of the mean score. Actually, 95% of scores lie within 1.96 standard deviations from the mean score – a figure which has great importance in inferential statistics.

KEY POINTS

- To describe nominal data, simply give the number or proportion in each category.
- To describe ordinal data or skewed data, use the median and range.
- To describe interval or ratio data which are normally distributed, use the mean and standard deviation.
- A fixed proportion of scores lie between each standard deviation and the mean for data which are normally distributed, but not for other data.

FURTHER READING

1. Clegg, F. *Simple Statistics*. (1982; Cambridge: Cambridge University Press.
2. Gardner, M. J., Altman, D. G. *Statistics with Confidence*. 1989; British Medical Journal, London.

Chapter Seven

Basic parametric statistics

Amanda J. Farrin

INTRODUCTION

The purpose of this chapter is to describe some basic statistical parametric tests, including the background, general structure and methods of calculation. It is important, when planning research studies, to consider both methods of data collection and data analysis. Therefore, knowledge of which statistical test is appropriate to individual study designs is vital. In this chapter we will consider how research *hypotheses* can be investigated through the use of statistical tests.

Often the research hypothesis involves some claim about a population *parameter*:

Examples

- 'At least half the work force in the clinic is in favour of new working conditions.'
- 'The national *prevalence* of schizophrenia in men is 15%.'
- The new treatment reduces the *incidence* of side-effects.'

Each of these statements can be treated as a *hypothesis.* In order to make decisions, it is necessary to test these hypotheses. In some situations it may be possible to look at the whole population concerned (e.g. the whole work force in the clinic) to determine the validity of these statements. In many situations this is not practicable (time, cost, etc.) and only a sample from the population will be available.

If only a sample is available, the sample mean will vary from sample to sample. How then can a hypothesis about the true population mean be tested when we cannot be sure whether the sample mean used to test it reflects it accurately? The way forward is to use the sampling distributions of means, which leads on to hypothesis (or significance) testing.

Statistical methods are often based on making assumptions, for example that the observed data are a sample from a population that is distributed in a particular way. The tests considered in this chapter are concerned with testing statistics, such as the mean, which requires an *interval* or *ratio* scale of measurement. In addition, the tests also involve assumptions that the data are *normally* distributed. Such tests are called *parametric tests.*

How can we judge if the data are normally distributed? The most simple or subjective approach is to look at a histogram of the data, which will clearly demonstrate if the data are obviously non-normal.[1] This approach is not so helpful in more borderline situations.

Sometimes when analysing data, it is not reasonable to assume that the data are normally distributed. In such situations, distribution-free or *non-parametric* statistical methods can be used. These tests can be used with *nominal* and *ordinal* data and make no assumptions of normality. These methods are discussed in more detail in Chapter 8.

An alternative to using non-parametric tests for non-normal data is to *transform* the data. Bland and Altman[2] give an introductory discussion of transforming data.

GENERAL STRUCTURE OF A STATISTICAL TEST

It is important to have an understanding of the general structure of a statistical test, which can be broken down into four steps.

Step 1: state the null and alternative hypotheses

- The *null hypothesis* (often denoted by H_0) is a statement of the simplest model that we are prepared to accept until sufficient evidence accrues to reject it. (For example, two treatments are equally effective.)
- The *alternative hypothesis* (often denoted by H_1) covers the alternatives we are interested in investigating and it usually covers all other possibilities. (For example, the two treatments are not equally effective, without specifying which one works best.)

Step 2: define and evaluate a test statistic

The general form of the *test statistic* is expressed in terms of the observed value of interest (e.g. the sample mean) and the value expected if the null hypothesis were true:

$$\text{test statistic} = \frac{\text{observed value} - \text{expected value}}{\text{standard error of observed value}}$$

Step 3: calculate the *P*-value

- The *P*-value can be thought of as a way to summarize what the data say about the credibility of the null hypothesis. It is the probability of observing a value of the test statistic at least as extreme as the value actually obtained from the data, assuming that the null hypothesis is true. So it is the probability of the observed result, or one more extreme, if the null hypothesis were true.

- The *P*-value is not the same as the probability that the null hypothesis is true.

Step 4: interpret the results

- This is a crucial stage of the process, so it is important to have a clear idea of how to interpret *P*-values.
- Since the *P*-value is a probability, it must lie between 0 (no chance) and 1 (absolutely certain). If the *P*-value is large (say, greater than 0.2), then the data have provided no evidence against the null hypothesis. If on the other hand, the *P*-value is very small (say less than 0.001), then the data provide convincing evidence against the null hypothesis. Between these two extremes, more cautious interpretation of *P*-values is required. Table 7.1 gives some guidance on interpreting *P*-values.

Table 7.1 *The interpretation of P-values*

***P*-value**	**Possible interpretation**
Between 0.1 and 1.0	Result consistent with H_0/H_0 is plausible (but not necessarily true)
Between 0.1 and 0.05	Result consistent with H_0/slight statistical evidence against H_0
Between 0.05 and 0.01	Some evidence against H_0
Between 0.01 and 0.001	Strong evidence against H_0
Between 0.001 and 0.0001	Very strong evidence against H_0
Less than 0.0001	H_0 cannot be believed

H_0 = the null hypothesis.

Remember:

- Evidence consistent with H_0 does not mean that the null hypothesis is true. It can be demonstrated to be false but rarely can it be proved true.
- A non-significant difference is not necessarily the same thing as no difference.
- A significant difference is not necessarily the same thing as an interesting or clinically relevant difference.
- If the *P*-value obtained is less than 0.05, the result is described as statistically significant at the 5% level. Even if a *P*-value is very small, this alone tells us nothing about the magnitude of the difference between two treatments.

Clinical significance is concerned with whether any difference between the two treatments is large enough to be of clinical relevance. For example, there may be a statistically significant difference in the effect of two drugs on blood pressure, one reducing it by an extra mmHg on average. This, however, is not of clinical significance as it would not influence any symptoms of high blood pressure.

Having carried out a hypothesis test and found evidence against the null hypothesis, it is then important to examine the data and usually a good idea to calculate a *confidence interval.*

Summary points

- A *P*-value is not the probability that the null hypothesis is true.
- A *P*-value is not necessarily large for small studies – it will depend on the size of the difference observed.
- A *P*-value is the probability of finding the observed result, or one more extreme if the null hypothesis is true.
- A *P*-value does not take only a limited number of values such as 0.1, 0.05. A *P*-value can take any value between zero and one and should be quoted in full if possible (e.g. $P = 0.0099$).

SETTING UP HYPOTHESES

Examples:

1. Consider patients completing a battery of tests. Of critical importance in costing is the average time taken to undertake the tests. A certain type of test has always been assumed to take 5 minutes. You want to test this hypothesis; you have no idea what the true value is.

   Step 1: state the null and the alternative hypotheses:

   - First, the null hypothesis must be set up: H_0: $\mu = 5$ minutes
     This states that the true mean (μ) for the population is 5 minutes.
   - The alternative hypothesis is: H_1: $\mu \neq 5$ minutes
     This is a two-sided alternative as it states that the true mean is not equal to five minutes, it could be greater or smaller than five minutes.

2. Suppose it is claimed that in a very large batch of instruments, no more than 10% of items contain some form of defect. To test this assertion:

   - First, the null hypothesis must be set up: H_0: $P = 0.1$
     This assumes that the true proportion of defectives is 10% or less.
   - The alternative hypothesis is: H_1: $P > 0.1$
     This is a one-sided alternative as it states that the true proportion of defectives is greater than 10%.

For further discussion of one- and two-sided tests read Bland and Altman.[3]

Having formally set up the hypotheses, the next step is to take a *random sample* from the population, obtain the sample statistic of interest (usually the mean), calculate the test statistic and see whether this supports the null hypothesis or not. The next three sections describe how and when to use three of the most common parametric statistical tests.

ONE SAMPLE *t*-TEST

Why use this test? We may wish to compare measurements made on a single group of patients to a reference value such as that for the general population.

Example:

In a study to examine actual energy intake compared with the recommended daily intake, the average daily energy intake (kJ) over 10 days was calculated for 11 clinically depressed patients.

The results are shown below:

5260	6805
5470	7515
5640	7515
6180	8230
6390	8770
6515	

The mean daily energy intake for the group as a whole is 6753.6 kJ
The standard deviation of these measurements is 1142.1 kJ

Looking at the data it can be seen that on average these patients had a daily energy intake below the recommended level of 7725 kJ, the average deficit being 971.4 kJ (7725 – 6753.6 kJ). To determine whether this difference is statistically significant, the one-sample *t*-test can be used to compare the energy intake of this sample of patients with the recommended daily intake of 7725 kJ.

Step 1: state the null and the alternative hypotheses:
Set up null and alternative hypotheses:
H_0: true mean = 7725 kJ
H_1: true mean $\neq$ 7725 kJ

Step 2: define and evaluate a test statistic:
You do not need to be able to do this test manually. For this and the following tests a computer can carry out the test rapidly and reliably. The

following description will help you to understand the rationale of the process and help you make sense of the findings.

For a one-sample *t*-test, the test statistic is denoted by *t*, as shown below:

$$t = \frac{\text{sample mean} - \text{hypothesized mean}}{\text{standard error of sample mean}}$$

$$\text{So } t = \frac{6753.6 - 7725}{1142.1/\sqrt{11}}$$

$$\text{So } t = -2.821$$

Now we need to use statistical tables of the *t distribution* to find the *P*-value associated with the observed value of *t*. The tables are included in Table 7.4 in the Appendix at the end of this chapter. The number of *degrees of freedom* is equal to the sample size minus one, so in this case, the number of degrees of freedom is 10 (11 – 1). For a two-sided test we ignore the sign and look for the largest tabulated value of *t* below our observed value in the row for 10 degrees of freedom.

From Table 7.4 we find that the *P*-value lies between 0.02 and 0.01.

This *P*-value indicates that the probability of obtaining a sample mean as small or smaller than 6753.6 kJ, if the true mean were 7725 kJ, is small. So we can conclude that there is strong statistical evidence to reject the null hypothesis (i.e. that the dietary intake of the 11 patients is significantly different to the recommended level of 7725 kJ).

The level of the *P*-value, however, gives no information about the magnitude of the difference in energy intake between this sample of patients and the recommended daily intake, nor about the uncertainty of the estimate of the difference. For this a *confidence interval* is needed. When presenting research results, it is important to show confidence intervals in addition to *P*-values.[3,4,5]

TWO SAMPLE *t*-TEST

When to use this test? When measurements are made on two different groups of subjects.

Why use this test? To assess the statistical significance of differences between two groups.

What sort of data are appropriate? Two independent groups of data.

Example:

In another study, the 24 hour total energy intake (MJ/day) was calculated for two groups of women suspected of having an eating disorder: a treatment group (receiving therapy sessions) and a control group. The results are shown in Table 7.2.

Table 7.2 *Energy intake in control and treatment groups*

	Control (n_1 = 13)	Treatment (n_2 = 9)
	6.13	8.79
	7.05	9.19
	7.48	9.21
	7.48	9.68
	7.53	9.69
	7.58	9.97
	7.90	11.51
	8.08	11.85
	8.09	12.79
	8.11	
	8.40	
	10.15	
	10.88	
Mean	8.066 MJ	10.298 MJ
SD	1.238	1.398

Looking at the group means, it can be seen that the treatment group has on average a higher energy intake than the control group, the average difference being 2.232 MJ/day. To assess the statistical significance of this difference the two-sample *t*-test can be used as it will compare the mean energy intake in the two groups.

Step 1: state the null and the alternative hypotheses:

- Set up null and alternative hypotheses:
  H_0: control group mean – treatment group mean = 0
  H_1: control group mean – treatment group mean ≠ 0

Step 2: define and evaluate a test statistic:
For a two-sample *t*-test, the test statistic, *t* is calculated as shown below:

$$t = \frac{\text{mean of group 1 (controls)} - \text{mean of group 2 (treatment)}}{\text{standard error of the difference in means}}$$

or

$$t = \frac{\bar{x}_1 - \bar{x}_2}{s.e.\ (\bar{x}_1 - \bar{x}_2)}$$

To calculate the standard error of the difference in the sample means, we need to first calculate the pooled standard deviation, *s*:

$$s = \sqrt{\frac{(n_1 - 1)s_1^2 + (n_2 - 1)s_2^2}{n_1 + n_2 - 2}}$$

where n_1 = sample size of control group; n_2 = sample size in treatment group and s_1 = standard deviation in control group; s_2 = standard deviation in treatment group:

$$s = \sqrt{\frac{12 \times 1.238^2 + 8 \times 1.398^2}{20}}$$

Then we have

s = 1.3044 MJ/day

$$s.e.\ (\bar{x}_1 - \bar{x}_2) = s \times \sqrt{\frac{1}{n_1} + \frac{1}{n_2}}$$

$$s.e.\ (\bar{x}_1 - \bar{x}_2) = 1.3044 \times \sqrt{\frac{1}{13} + \frac{1}{9}} = 0.5656 \text{ MJ/day}$$

So the test statistic is:

$$t = \frac{8.066 - 10.298}{0.5656} = -3.95$$

Now we need to use statistical tables (t-distribution) to find the P-value associated with the observed value of t (Table 7.4). In this case, the number of degrees of freedom is equal to the sum of the two sample sizes minus two, so in this case, the number of degrees of freedom is 20 (13 + 9 – 2). For a two-sided test we can ignore the sign and look for the largest tabulated value of t below our observed value in the row of 20 degrees of freedom.

From Table 7.4 we find that the P-value is less than 0.001.

This P-value indicates that the probability of obtaining a difference in means as large or larger than 2.232 MJ/day, if the true difference were zero, is almost zero. We can conclude that there is very strong evidence to reject the null hypothesis, (i.e. that there is a statistically significant difference in the total energy expenditure of the treatment group compared with the control group). Again it is useful to also calculate confidence intervals.

As a rough guide when using t-tests, if the sample size is larger than 30, tables of the normal distribution (Tables 7.5a and b) can be used, rather than the t distribution.

PAIRED *t*-TEST

When to use this test? When two measurements have been made on each subject in a group – usually once before and once after treatment or intervention. The difference between the measurements can be calculated for each subject and the mean difference can be calculated for the group of subjects.

Why use this test? To assess the statistical significance of the average effect of treatment on a single group of subjects.

What sort of data are appropriate? Paired data (for instance, 'before and after' measurements on the same set of patients or measurements on patients and individually matched healthy controls).

Example:
In an observational study, the average (mean) daily dietary intake was calculated for 11 women over 10 pre-menstrual and 10 post-menstrual days. The data are summarized in Table 7.3.

We are interested in the average differences between the observations for each individual and the variability of these differences (i.e. *within subject differences* not between subject differences). Looking at the data, it can be seen that dietary intake is lower post-menstrually for all 11 women and the average difference is 1320.5 kJ. To assess whether this difference is statistically significant, the paired *t*-test can be used. The method is similar to the one-sample *t*-test as it treats the differences as if they were a single sample of observations.

Table 7.3 *Dietary intake in pre- and post-menstrual women*

Subject	Dietary intake (kJ)in pre-menstrual women	Dietary intake (kJ) in post-menstrual women	(pre–post) difference
1	5260	3910	1350
2	5475	4220	1250
3	5640	3885	1755
4	6180	5160	1020
5	6390	5645	745
6	6515	4680	1835
7	6805	5265	1540
8	7515	5975	1540
9	7515	6790	725
10	8230	6900	1330
11	8770	7335	1435
Mean	6753.6	5433.2	1320.5
SD	1142.1	1216.8	366.7

Step 1: set up null and alternative hypotheses:
H_0: $\bar{d} = 0$
H_1: $\bar{d} \neq 0$
$\bar{d}$ = mean of the differences

Step 2: define and evaluate a test statistic:
For a paired *t*-test, the test statistic, *t*, is calculated as:

$$t = \frac{\text{mean differences} - 0}{\text{standard error of mean difference}}$$

where standard error of mean difference = standard deviation of the differences divided by the square root of the sample size.

So

$$t = \frac{1320.5}{3.667/\sqrt{11}}$$

$$= 11.94$$

Now we need to use the statistical tables (Table 7.4) to find the *P*-value associated with the observed value of *t*. The number of degrees of freedom is equal to the sample size minus one, so in this case the number of degrees of freedom is 10 (11–1). For a two-sided test we ignore the sign and look for the largest tabulated value of *t* below our observed value in the row of 10 degrees of freedom.

From Table 7.4, we find that the *P*-value is very much less than 0.001. This *P*-value indicates that the probability of obtaining a difference as large or larger than 1320.5, if the true difference were zero, is almost zero. We can conclude that there is very strong evidence to reject the null hypothesis (i.e. that there is a statistically significant difference in the dietary intake energy intake in the pre-menstrual period compared with the post-menstrual period). Again it is useful to also calculate an appropriate confidence interval for the mean difference.

COMPUTER SOFTWARE

The previous sections have shown how to carry out several statistical tests using pen, paper and a calculator. Researchers with access to a computer, will find that most spreadsheet packages and all statistical packages have the capability to carry out these tests (and many more besides). Most packages will produce a test statistic (such as *t* or *z*), a *P*-value and a confidence interval, which the researcher needs to interpret in the same manner as described in this chapter.

Two of the more straightforward packages, which are easy to use are EXCEL (a spreadsheet package) and MINITAB (a statistical package). Other statistical packages such as SPSS for Windows are more sophisticated, offering a wealth of statistical techniques that often appear bewildering to the unfamiliar user.

CONCLUSIONS

When choosing an appropriate method of analysis think about:

- The number of groups of observations – one, two or more.
- Independent or dependent groups of observations – paired or unpaired data.
- The type of data – measurements, proportions, categorical data.
- The distribution of data – normal or not?
- The objective of the analysis – the research hypothesis will determine the analysis.

KEY POINTS

- The one- sample *t*-test can be used to assess the statistical significance of the difference between the mean of a sample of subjects and a population value.
- The two-sample *t*-test can be used to assess the statistical significance of the difference between the means of two groups of subjects.
- The paired *t*-test can be used to assess the statistical significance of the average effect of a drug or treatment on a single group of subjects.

REFERENCES

1. Altman, D. G., Bland, J. M. The normal distribution. *British Medical Journal,* 1995; **310**, 298.
2. Bland, J. M., Altman, D.G. The use of transformations when comparing two means. *British Medical Journal,* 1996; **312**, 1153.
3. Bland, J. M., Altman, D.G. One and two sided tests of significance. *British Medical Journal*, 1994; **309**, 248.
4. Swinscow, T. D. V. (revised:Campbell, M. J.) *Statistics at Square One.* 1996; BMJ Publishing Group, London.
5. Gardner, M. J., Altman, D. G. (eds). *Statistics with Confidence.* 1989; BMJ Publishing Group, London.
6. Altman, D. G. *Practical Statistics for Medical Research.* 1996; Chapman & Hall, London.

APPENDIX

Table 7.4 *t Distribution*

Degrees of freedom	Two-tailed probability (*P*) 0.2	0.1	0.05	0.02	0.01	0.001
1	3.078	6.314	12.706	31.821	63.657	636.619
2	1.886	2.920	4.303	6.965	9.925	31.599
3	1.638	2.353	3.182	4.541	5.841	12.924
4	1.533	2.132	2.776	3.747	4.604	8.610
5	1.476	2.015	2.571	3.365	4.032	6.869
6	1.440	1.943	2.447	3.143	3.707	5.959
7	1.415	1.895	2.365	2.998	3.499	5.408
8	1.397	1.860	2.306	2.896	3.355	4.041
9	1.383	1.833	2.262	2.821	3.250	4.781
10	1.372	1.812	2.228	2.764	3.169	4.587
11	1.363	1.796	2.201	2.718	3.106	4.437
12	1.356	1.782	2.179	2.681	3.055	4.318
13	1.350	1.771	2.160	2.650	3.012	4.221
14	1.350	1.761	2.145	2.624	2.977	4.140
15	1.341	1.753	2.131	2.602	2.947	4.073
16	1.337	1.746	2.120	2.583	2.921	4.015
17	1.333	1.740	2.110	2.567	2.898	3.965
18	1.330	1.734	2.101	2.552	2.878	3.922
19	1.328	1.729	2.093	2.539	2.861	3.883
20	1.325	1.725	2.086	2.528	2.845	3.850
21	1.323	1.721	2.080	2.518	2.831	3.819
22	1.321	1.717	2.074	2.508	2.819	3.792
23	1.319	1.714	2.069	2.500	2.807	3.768
24	1.318	1.711	2.064	2.492	2.797	3.745
25	1.316	1.708	2.060	2.485	2.787	3.725
26	1.315	1.706	2.056	2.479	2.779	3.707
27	1.314	1.703	2.052	2.473	2.771	3.690
28	1.313	1.701	2.048	2.467	2.763	3.674
29	1.311	1.699	2.045	2.462	2.756	3.659
30	1.310	1.697	2.042	2.457	2.750	3.646
31	1.309	1.696	2.040	2.453	2.744	3.633
32	1.309	1.694	2.037	2.449	2.738	3.622
33	1.308	1.692	2.035	2.445	2.733	3.611
34	1.307	1.691	2.032	2.441	2.728	3.601
35	1.306	1.690	2.030	2.438	2.724	3.591
36	1.306	1.688	2.028	2.434	2.719	3.582
37	1.305	1.687	2.026	2.431	2.715	3.574
38	1.304	1.686	2.024	2.429	2.712	3.566
39	1.304	1.685	2.023	2.426	2.708	3.558

►

40	1.303	1.684	2.021	2.423	2.704	3.551
41	1.303	1.683	2.020	2.421	2.701	3.544
42	1.302	1.682	2.018	2.418	2.698	3.538
43	1.302	1.681	2.017	2.416	2.695	3.532
44	1.301	1.680	2.015	2.414	2.692	3.526
45	1.301	1.679	2.014	2.412	2.690	3.520
46	1.300	1.679	2.013	2.410	2.687	3.515
47	1.300	1.678	2.012	2.408	2.685	3.510
48	1.299	1.677	2.011	2.407	2.682	3.505
49	1.299	1.677	2.010	2.405	2.680	3.500
50	1.299	1.676	2.009	2.403	2.678	3.496
60	1.296	1.671	2.000	2.390	2.660	3.460
70	1.294	1.667	1.994	2.381	2.648	3.435
80	1.292	1.664	1.990	2.374	2.639	3.416
90	1.291	1.662	1.987	2.368	2.632	3.402
100	1.290	1.660	1.984	2.364	2.626	3.390

Example: For an observed test statistic $t = 2.11$, with 16 degrees of freedom, we have $0.05 < P < 0.1$

Table 7.5a *Normal distribution (two tailed)*

z	*P*	*z*	*P*	*z*	*P*	*z*	*P*
0.00	1.0000						
0.05	0.9601	1.05	0.2937	2.05	0.0404	3.10	0.00194
0.10	0.9203	1.10	0.2713	2.10	0.0357	3.20	0.00137
0.15	0.8808	1.15	0.2501	2.15	0.0316	3.30	0.00097
0.20	0.8415	1.20	0.2301	2.20	0.0278	3.40	0.00067
0.25	0.8026	1.25	0.2113	2.25	0.0244	3.50	0.00047
0.30	0.7642	1.30	0.1936	2.30	0.0214	3.60	0.00032
0.35	0.7263	1.35	0.1770	2.35	0.0188	3.70	0.00022
0.40	0.6892	1.40	0.1615	2.40	0.0164	3.80	0.00014
0.45	0.6527	1.45	0.1471	2.45	0.0143	3.90	0.00010
0.50	0.6171	1.50	0.1336	2.50	0.0124	4.00	0.00006
0.55	0.5823	1.55	0.1211	2.55	0.0108		
0.60	0.5485	1.60	0.1096	2.60	0.0093		
0.65	0.5157	1.65	0.0989	2.65	0.0080		
0.70	0.4839	1.70	0.0891	2.70	0.0069		
0.75	0.4533	1.75	0.0801	2.75	0.0060		
0.80	0.4237	1.80	0.0719	2.80	0.0051		
0.85	0.3953	1.85	0.0643	2.85	0.0044		
0.90	0.3681	1.90	0.0574	2.90	0.0037		
0.95	0.3421	1.95	0.0512	2.95	0.0032		
1.00	0.3173	2.00	0.0455	3.00	0.0027		

Example: The two-tailed *P*-value for an observed test statistic (z) of 2.10 is 0.0357

Table 7.5b *Normal distribution (two tailed) – standard normal deviates*

P **(two-tailed *P*-values)**	***z*** **standard normal deviates**
1.0	0.000
0.9	0.126
0.8	0.253
0.7	0.385
0.6	0.524
0.5	0.674
0.4	0.842
0.3	1.036
0.2	1.282
0.1	1.645
0.05	1.960
0.02	2.326
0.01	2.576
0.001	3.291
0.0001	3.891

Example: For an observed test statistic $z = 2.11$, we have $P < 0.05$

Chapter Eight

Basic non-parametric statistics

Amanda J. Farrin

INTRODUCTION

The purpose of this chapter is to describe some basic statistical non-parametric tests, including the background, methods of calculation and situations in which such tests are appropriate. It is important, when planning research studies, to consider both methods of data collection and data analysis and a knowledge of which statistical test is appropriate to individual study designs is vital. This chapter will consider how to use a variety of non-parametric statistical tests.

The assumption of *Normality* underlies many statistical tests, such as *t*-tests, as detailed in Chapter 7. When analysing data using such tests, it is assumed the data are drawn from Normal populations. The validity of any conclusions from such analyses depends (to some extent) on the validity of these assumptions.

It is not always correct to assume that the data are drawn from a Normal population. The distribution of the sample of data may show marked skewedness or asymmetry. It is therefore useful to construct statistical tests which are less restrictive and make weaker assumptions about the underlying distribution of the data. These are known as *non-parametric tests*.

In practice we usually only perform one analysis of a data set choosing between parametric and non-parametric methods. It is usual to use a parametric method, unless there is a clear indication that it is not valid. Situations where a non-parametric test *might* be appropriate include:

- Non-normal or skewed data.
- Small samples.
- Ordinal data.

It is important to realize that if we apply different tests to the same data then we do not expect them to give the same answer, but in general two valid methods will give similar answers. Non-parametric tests:

- Are less powerful than the equivalent parametric test (especially in small samples) and

- Tend to give a less significant (larger) *P*-value.

Non-parametric tests are usually based on order statistics and ranks. When the observations are arranged in increasing order of size, they are known as *order statistics,* while the places of the observations in this order are known as *ranks.*

Example:

Score	7	9	10	12	12	9	12	11	–13
Observation	x_1	x_2	x_3	x_4	x_5	x_6	x_7	x_8	x_9
Score	–13	7	9	9	10	11	12	12	12
Order statistics	$x_{(1)}$	$x_{(2)}$	$x_{(3)}$	$x_{(4)}$	$x_{(5)}$	$x_{(6)}$	$x_{(7)}$	$x_{(8)}$	$x_{(9)}$
Ranks	1	2	3.5	5	6	8	8	8	

In this example, some of the observations take the same value, for instance x_2 and x_6 both take the value of 9 while x_4, x_5 and x_7 all take the value 12. In order to assign ranks to these *tied* observations, first imagine that they take slightly different values, for instance x_2 and x_6 take the values 8.9 and 9.1, these values would then be given the ranks 3 and 4. Secondly, calculate the average of these ranks (3.5) and assign it to the observations x_2 and x_6.

Shown below is the general structure of a *hypothesis test* as outlined in Chapter 7. These four steps should be followed for all non-parametric analyses:

1. State the null and alternative hypotheses.
2. Define and evaluate a test statistic.
3. Calculate the *P*-value.
4. Interpret the results.

Table 8.1 below gives some guidance on interpreting *P*-values:

Table 8.1 *Interpretation of P-values*

***P*-value**	**Possible interpretation**
Between 0.1 and 1.0	Result consistent with H_0/H_0 is plausible (but not necessarily true)
Between 0.1 and 0.05	Result consistent with H_0/slight statistical evidence against H_0
Between 0.05 and 0.01	Some evidence against H_0
Between 0.01 and 0.001	Strong evidence against H_0
Between 0.001 and 0.0001	Very strong evidence against H_0
Less than 0.0001	H_0 cannot be believed

H_0 = the null hypothesis

When choosing methods of analysis, the following issues should be considered:

- Number of groups of observations – This chapter and Chapter 7 describe statistical methods appropriate for analysing one or two groups of data. More complicated methods are required for more than two groups. The latter include the analysis of variance (ANOVA – a parametric test) or the Kruskal-Wallis test (a non-parametric equivalent to the ANOVA again used for situations with more than two groups of data), Altman and Bland[1] give an illustration of ANOVA.
- Independent (unpaired) or dependent (paired) groups of observations – For dependent groups, a paired test is appropriate. This would be used in cases where test subjects are either matched in some way or are compared with themselves (e.g. before and after starting a medication). In contrast, some experiments analyse independent (or unpaired) groups (i.e. un-matched or different test subjects).
- The type of data and the distribution of data – The type and distribution of the data will help determine whether a parametric or non-parametric approach should be employed (see Chapter 7).

The next three sections describe how and when to use some of the most common non-parametric tests.

WILCOXON SIGNED RANK SUM TEST

This can be thought of as the non-parametric equivalent of the one sample *t*-test.

- Why use this test? When comparing data from a single group of subjects to a reference value, but the assumptions behind the one sample *t*-test are violated.

Example: (refer to the example for the one sample t-test in Chapter 7). In this study a second group of 11 patients (with chronic fatigue syndrome – CFS) were also studied. Their average daily energy intake (kJ) over 10 days was calculated in order to compare it with the recommended daily intake of 7725 kJ. Table 8.2 shows the results.

Step 1: set up null (H_0) and alternative (H_1) hypotheses:

H_0: The recommended daily intake is 7726 kJ (or in strict statistical terms that the location for the distribution is 7725 kJ).

H_1: The location for the distribution is not 7725 kJ.

Table 8.2 *Results of the CFS study*

Subject no.	Daily energy intake (kJ)	Difference from 7725 kJ	Ranks of absolute differences	Sign
1	6265	1460	9.5	+
2	6265	1460	9.5	+
3	6560	1165	8	+
4	6610	1115	7	+
5	7130	595	5	+
6	7415	310	4	+
7	7580	145	3	+
8	7715	10	1	+
9	7850	–125	2	–
10	8325	–600	6	–
11	9770	–2045	11	–

Step 2: define and evaluate a test statistic:
In most cases, you will simply use a computerized statistical package. The following step-by-step approach will help you to understand this process:

Test statistic = $W = \min\{W_+, W_-\}$

where W_+ = sum of the ranks for positive differences = 47
and W_- = sum of the ranks for negative differences = 19

The minimum of these gives the test statistic *W*

$$\text{So } W = \min\{W_+, W_-\} = 19$$

Now we need to use Table 8.5 in the Appendix at the end of the chapter to find the *P*-value associated with the observed value of W. In this case, the sample size is 11, so we look for the value of W in the row for n = 11. From the Table, it can be seen that $W = 19$ is greater than the values of *W* for *P*-values of 5% and 1%, so in this case the *P*-value is greater than 0.05 (or 5%).

We can conclude that there is no statistical evidence to reject the null hypothesis (i.e. this sample of patients provides no statistical evidence that the daily energy intake of CFS patients is any different to the recommended level of 7725 kJ).

Summary of the procedure

- Calculate the difference between each observation and the value of interest.
- Ignoring the signs of the differences, rank them in order of size.
- Calculate the sum of the ranks of all the negative (or positive) ranks

corresponding to the observations below (or above) the chosen hypothesised value.

Note: In some cases differences of 0 will be observed – ignore these completely and base the test on the number, n, of *non-zero* differences.

MANN-WHITNEY U TEST (ALSO KNOWN AS THE WILCOXON RANK SUM TEST)

This can be thought of as the non-parametric equivalent of the two sample t-test.

- When to use this test? When measurements are collected on two different groups of subjects and assumptions behind the two sample t-test are violated.
- Why use this test? To assess the statistical significance of differences between two groups.

Example: (refer to the example for the two sample t-test in Chapter 7). When analysing the results in this study (the effects of treatment on the 24-hour total energy intake (MJ/day) in women with eating disorders), it was decided that a non-parametric analysis would be more appropriate as the sample size was small and the distribution of the data looked skewed. The data from the two groups are shown in Table 8.3, together with the accompanying ranks. All 22 observations were ranked from lowest to highest, ignoring which group each observation belonged to.

Table 8.3 *Results of the eating disorders study*

Control group (n_1 = 13)	Ranks	Treatment group (n_2 = 9)	Ranks
6.13	1	8.79	12
7.05	2	9.19	13
7.48	3.5	9.21	14
7.48	3.5	9.68	15
7.53	5	9.69	16
7.58	6	9.97	17
7.90	7	11.51	20
8.08	8	11.85	21
8.09	9	12.79	22
8.11	10		
8.40	11		
10.15	18		
10.88	19		
Total	103		150

Step 1: set up null (H_0) and alternative (H_1) hypotheses:
H_0 : The location for each group is the same (i.e. there are no differences between the results of the control and treatment groups).

H_1 : The location for each group is not the same (i.e. there is a difference between the results of the control and treatment groups).

If H_0 is true there should be no pattern to the ranks allocated to each group.

In practice you would use a computer to produce this result. The following is shown to help you understand the process of analysing ranked data.

Step 2: define and evaluate a test statistic:

Test statistic = U = min $\{U_1, U_2\}$

U_1 and U_2 are calculated using R_1 (sum of the ranks for group 1) and R_2 (sum of the ranks for group 2)

$$\text{So} \quad R_1 = 103 \quad \text{and} \quad R_2 = 150$$

U_1 and U_2 can then be calculated using the following formulae:

$$U_1 = R_1 - \frac{n_1(n_1 + 1)}{2} = 103 - \frac{13 \times 14}{2}$$

$$U_2 = R_2 - \frac{n_2(n_2 + 1)}{2} = 150 - \frac{9 \times 10}{2}$$

$$\text{Thus } U_1 = 12 \text{ and } U_2 = 105$$

The arithmetic can be checked using the formula: $U_2 = n_1 n_2 - U_1$
So in this case: $n_1 n_2 - U_1 = 13 \times 9 - 12 = 117 - 12 = 105 = U_2$
So the test statistic, U = min $\{U_1, U_2\} = 12$

Now we need to use Tables 8.7 and 8.8 in the Appendix at the end of the chapter to find the *P*-value associated with the observed value U = 12. In this case, the sample sizes of the two groups are 13 and 9, so $n_L = 13$ and $n_S = 9$. We look along the row for $n_L = 13$ and down the column for $n_S = 9$. These coincide at 28 (5% significance level – Table 8.7) and at 20 (1% significance level – Table 8.8). So from the Tables, it can be seen that U = 12 is less than the values of W for *P*-values of 5% and 1%, so the *P*-value is less than 0.01 (or 1%).

We can conclude that there is strong statistical evidence to reject the null hypothesis (i.e. this sample of patients provides strong statistical evidence that the total energy intake is different in the treatment group compared to the control group).

WILCOXON SIGNED RANK TEST (FOR PAIRED DATA)

This can be thought of as the non-parametric equivalent of the paired *t*-test.

When to use this test? When two measurements are made on each subject in a group or when measurements are made on a group of patients and individually matched controls; and the assumptions behind the paired *t*-test are violated.

Why use this test? To assess the statistical significance of the average effect of treatment on a single group of subjects or two groups of matched subjects.

Example:

In a cross-over study, 10 patients received drug A for 10 days and a placebo for 10 days. The order in which the drug and placebo was given to each patient was determined at random. Each patient's anxiety score were recorded at the end of each 10-day period. The results are shown in Table 8.4. The difference between the anxiety scores for the drug and placebo period is calculated and the rank of the difference (ignoring the sign) is determined.

Table 8.4 *Anxiety scores in active drug and placebo groups*

Subject	Drug A anxiety score (0–30)	Placebo anxiety score (0–30)	Difference	Absolute difference	Rank	Sign
1	19	22	–3	3	6.5	–
2	11	15	–4	4	8	–
3	14	17	–3	3	6.5	–
4	17	19	–2	2	5	–
5	23	22	1	1	2.5	+
6	11	12	–1	1	2.5	–
7	15	14	1	1	2.5	+
8	19	11	8	8	10	+
9	11	17	–6	6	9	–
10	8	7	1	1	2.5	+

Step 1: set up null (H_0) and alternative (H_1) hypotheses:

H_0: The location for the distribution of the differences is zero (i.e. there is no difference between the anxiety scores on drug A and placebo).

H_1: The location for the distribution of the differences is not zero (i.e. there is a difference between the anxiety scores on drug A and placebo).

Step 2: define and evaluate a test statistic:
Again, you would use a computer to analyse these data. In this case:

Test statistic = W = min $\{W_+, W_-\}$

W_+ = Sum of the ranks for positive differences = 17.5
W_- = Sum of the ranks for negative differences = 37.5

$$\text{So } W = \min\{W_+, W_-\} = 17.5$$

Now we need to use Table 8.5 in the Appendix at the end of the chapter to find the *P*-value associated with the observed value of W. In this case, the sample size is 10, so we look for the value of W in the row for $n = 10$. From the Table, it can be seen that W = 17.5 is greater than the values of W for *P*-values of 5% and 1%, so the *P*-value is greater than 0.05 (or 5%).

We can conclude that there is no statistical evidence to reject the null hypothesis (i.e. there is no statistical evidence that there are differences in patient anxiety levels when comparing drug A to a placebo).

COMPUTER SOFTWARE

The previous sections have shown how easy it is to carry out non-parametric statistical tests using pen, paper and a calculator, however this is a methodical process which takes time. Researchers with access to a computer will normally wish to use a spreadsheet package or a statistical package to carry out the 'number crunching', especially if many analyses are undertaken.

- Most statistical packages (such as MINITAB, SPSS) contain a range of non-parametric procedures and will be able to produce a test statistic (such as U or W), a *P*-value and possibly, a confidence interval, which the researcher needs to interpret.
- Some packages routinely use a large sample approximation for non-parametric tests, regardless of sample size, so it would be wise to check the computer output carefully, particularly for small samples, (for instance, samples of less than 30) otherwise errors of interpretation may occur.
- Spreadsheet packages, such as EXCEL, very rarely contain non-parametric techniques as standard, however it is possible to write macros for some non-parametric techniques.
- Statistical 'add on packages' are available commercially which allow several spreadsheets to carry out more sophisticated statistical calculations.

PLANNING STUDIES

The method of analysing data should be appropriate for each set of data. Non-parametric methods are sometimes chosen because the sample size is small. When planning a study, an appropriate sample size should be calculated at the same time as decisions regarding data collection and methods of analyses. Sample size calculations are sometimes complex and depend on the method of analysis. The calculations involve:

- The variability of the outcome measure in the study population.
- The significance level required.
- The smallest clinically worthwhile effect and the statistical power (that is, the chance of detecting a clinically worthwhile effect if one exists).

For details of how to carry out a power calculation refer to Campbell *et al.*[2] and Day and Graham.[3] Machin and Campbell[4] provide comprehensive tables for sample size calculations.

CONCLUSIONS

As with all significance tests remember that a non-significant difference is not necessarily the same thing as no difference and a significant difference is not necessarily the same thing as an interesting or clinically relevant difference.

When choosing an appropriate method of analysis think about:

- The number of groups of observations – one, two or more.
- Independent or dependent groups of observations – paired or unpaired data.
- The type of data – measurements, proportions, categorical data.
- The distribution of data – normal or not?
- The choice of whether to use a parametric or non-parametric test will depend on the sample size, data type, and the distribution of data.
- The objective of the analysis – the research hypothesis will determine the analysis.

KEY POINTS

- The Wilcoxon signed rank sum test can be used to assess the statistical significance of the difference between a sample of subjects and a population value.
- The Mann-Whitney U test (or Wilcoxon rank sum test) can be used to assess the statistical significance of the difference between two

independent groups of subjects and may be thought of as the non-parametric equivalent of an unpaired *t*-test.

- The Wilcoxon signed rank test can also be used to assess the statistical significance of the average effect of a treatment on a single group of subjects or the difference between a group of patients and individually matched controls and may be thought of as the non-parametric equivalent of a paired *t*-test.

REFERENCES

1. Altman, D. G., Bland, J. M. Comparing several groups using analysis of variance. *British Medical Journal*, 1996; **312**, 1472–3.
2. Campbell, M. J., Julious, S. A., Altman, D.G. Estimating samples sizes for binary, ordered categorical, and continuous outcomes in two group comparisons. *British Medical Journal*, 1995; **311**, 1145–8.
3. Day, S. J., Graham, D. F. Sample size and power for comparing two or more treatment groups in clinical trials. *British Medical Journal*, 1989; **299**, 663–5.
4. Machin, D., Campbell, M. J. *Statistical tables for design of clinical trials.* 1987; Blackwell Scientific, Oxford.

APPENDIX

Table 8.5 *Wilcoxon signed rank*

n	5%	1%	*n*	5%	1%
1	–	–	16	29	19
2	–	–	17	34	23
3	–	–	18	40	27
4	–	–	19	46	32
5	–	–	20	52	37
6	0	–	21	58	42
7	2	–	22	65	48
8	3	0	23	73	54
9	5	1	24	81	61
10	8	3	25	89	68
11	10	5	26	98	75
12	13	7	27	107	83
13	17	9	28	116	91
14	21	12	29	126	100
15	25	15	30	137	109

►

Table 8.5 (continued)

n	5%	1%	*n*	5%	1%
31	147	118	41	279	233
32	159	128	42	294	247
33	170	138	43	310	261
34	182	148	44	327	276
35	195	159	45	361	291
36	208	171	46	378	307
37	221	182	47	396	322
38	235	194	48	415	339
39	249	207	49	434	355
40	264	220	50	453	373

Table 8.6 Mann-Whitney, equal sample sizes

n	5%	1%	*n*	5%	1%
1	–	–	26	230	198
2	–	–	27	250	216
3	–	–	28	272	235
4	0	–	29	294	255
5	2	0	30	317	276
6	5	2	31	341	298
7	8	4	32	365	321
8	13	7	33	391	344
9	17	11	34	418	369
10	23	16	35	445	394
11	30	21	36	473	420
12	37	27	37	503	447
13	45	34	38	533	475
14	55	42	39	564	504
15	64	51	40	596	533
16	75	60	41	628	564
17	87	70	42	662	595
18	99	81	43	697	627
19	113	93	44	732	660
20	127	105	45	769	694
21	142	118	46	806	729
22	158	133	47	845	765
23	175	148	48	884	802
24	192	164	49	924	839
25	211	180	50	965	877

Table 8.7 Mann-Whitney, unequal sample sizes, 5% significance level

n_L \ n_S	2	3	4	5	6	7	8	9	10	11	12	13	14	15	16	17	18	19	20	21	22	23	24
2	–																						
3	–	–																					
4	–	–	–																				
5	–	0	1	–																			
6	–	1	2	3	–																		
7	–	1	3	5	6	–																	
8	0	2	4	6	8	10	–																
9	0	2	4	7	10	12	15	–															
10	0	3	5	8	11	14	17	20	–														
11	0	3	6	9	13	16	19	23	26	–													
12	1	4	7	11	14	18	22	26	29	33	–												
13	1	4	8	12	16	20	24	28	33	37	41	–											
14	1	5	9	13	17	22	26	31	36	40	45	50	–										
15	1	5	10	14	19	24	29	34	39	44	49	54	59	–									
16	1	6	11	15	21	26	31	37	42	47	53	59	64	70	–								
17	2	6	11	17	22	28	34	39	45	51	57	63	69	75	81	–							
18	2	7	12	18	24	30	36	42	48	55	61	67	74	80	86	93	–						
19	2	7	13	19	25	32	38	45	52	58	65	72	78	85	92	99	106	–					
20	2	8	14	20	27	34	41	48	55	62	69	76	83	90	98	105	112	119	–				
21	3	8	15	22	29	36	43	50	58	65	73	80	88	96	103	111	119	126	134	–			
22	3	9	16	23	30	38	45	53	61	69	77	85	93	101	109	117	125	133	141	150	–		
23	3	9	17	24	32	40	48	56	64	73	81	89	98	106	115	123	132	140	149	157	166	–	
24	3	10	17	25	33	45	50	59	67	76	85	94	102	111	120	129	138	147	156	165	174	183	–
25	3	10	18	27	35	44	53	62	71	80	89	98	107	117	126	135	145	154	163	173	182	192	201

Note : n_S is the sample size of the smaller group; n_L is the sample size of the larger group

Table 8.8 Mann-Whitney, unequal sample sizes, 1% significance level

n_L \ n_S	2	3	4	5	6	7	8	9	10	11	12	13	14	15	16	17	18	19	20	21	22	23	24
2	–																						
3	–	–																					
4	–	–	–																				
5	–	–	–	–																			
6	–	–	0	1	–																		
7	–	–	0	1	3	–																	
8	–	–	1	2	4	6	–																
9	–	0	1	3	5	7	9	–															
10	–	0	2	4	6	9	11	13	–														
11	–	0	2	5	7	10	13	16	18	–													
12	–	1	3	6	9	12	15	18	21	24	–												
13	–	1	3	7	10	13	17	20	24	27	31	–											
14	–	1	4	7	11	15	18	22	26	30	34	38	–										
15	–	2	5	8	12	16	20	24	29	33	37	42	46	–									
16	–	2	5	9	13	18	22	27	31	36	41	45	50	55	–								
17	–	2	6	10	15	19	24	29	34	39	44	49	54	60	65	–							
18	–	2	6	11	16	21	26	31	37	42	47	53	58	64	70	75	–						
19	0	3	7	12	17	22	28	33	39	45	51	57	63	69	74	81	87	–					
20	0	3	8	13	18	24	30	36	42	48	54	60	67	73	79	86	92	99	–				
21	0	3	8	14	19	25	32	38	44	51	58	64	71	78	84	91	98	105	112	–			
22	0	4	9	14	21	27	34	40	47	54	61	68	75	82	89	96	104	111	118	125	–		
23	0	4	9	15	22	29	35	43	50	57	64	72	79	87	94	102	109	117	125	132	140	–	
24	0	4	10	16	23	30	37	45	52	60	68	75	83	91	99	107	115	123	131	139	147	155	–
25	0	5	10	17	24	32	39	47	55	63	71	79	87	96	104	112	121	129	138	146	155	163	172

Note : n_S is the sample size of the smaller group; n_L is the sample size of the larger group.

Chapter Nine

Using computers to facilitate research

Patrick Harkin

INTRODUCTION

The increase in power and the reduction in costs of desk-top computers during the 1990s has resulted in a massive increase in their use in all fields of medical research. Computers have now a position in society equivalent to motorcars in the 1960s. Just as motor vehicles in pre-war Britain were expensive items operated by businesses as essentials or by individuals as luxury or hobby items before gaining wide acceptance, computers are now cheap, reliable, and accepted as normal practice. Early car owners knew their machines inside and out – in contrast a modern driver knows how to work his car and perform some simple maintenance tasks, but relies on professionals for support. In a similar way, we need to know how to work our computers, but do not need to know how they work!

As far as possible, this chapter has been kept jargon-free. A glossary of key computing terms is found at the end of this chapter.

WHAT ARE COMPUTERS?

One definition of a computer is *a versatile, programmable machine which:*

- Acquires and stores data.
- Allows the manipulation of that data.

All medical research contains areas in which one or more of these features of a computer can be of assistance. In addition, appropriate computer equipment eases communication between different people and provides a level of security for your work which is not easy to achieve using 'paper methods'.

Desktop computers are made up of several common components (Table 9.1). Almost all new machines on the market also feature *multimedia* options such as CD-ROM drives, (which are like audio CDs but can carry programmes, music and video), sound-cards and speakers.

Table 9.1 *Components of a standard desktop computer*

Component	Category	Function	Comment
Keyboard	Input device	Entry of text (including numbers)	Universal
Mouse	Input device	Interaction with on-screen display	Almost universal
Monitor (screen/ display)	Output device	Display of text or graphical output. Typical size 14 inches (35.5 cm). 15–17 inches (38–43 cm) are better particularly if the computer is used for multimedia applications (e.g. video games and CD-ROM materials)	Single most expensive component
Random access memory RAM	Storage device	Short-term memory store. Holds information on which the computer is currently working. This is the equivalent of 'working memory' in humans	Retains information only when the computer is powered. Measured in size using megabytes (MB)
Hard disk	Storage device	Permanently holds information (e.g. files/data)	Retains information even when switched off. Measured in gigabytes (GB)
Floppy disk	Storage device	Holds information, and can be moved from machine to machine. They act as a portable medium to allow the storage and transport of files and documents.	Much smaller capacity than the hard disk but useful for backup of files and transfer of data.

CHOOSING A COMPUTER

Do not rush out and purchase a new or second-hand computer and then ask yourself, 'How can I use this?' Instead, turn the problem around and ask yourself these questions:

- What tasks do I need to perform?
- What software* will I need to perform these tasks?
- What hardware† will I need to run this software?

If you answer each of these questions in turn, you will find the selection of the correct equipment much simpler and you will also reduce the risk of finding yourself with an expensive piece of obsolete equipment. Computer equipment depreciates very rapidly, therefore whenever you buy, you are likely to find the same or a better machine available for significantly less money within only 3 or 4 months. This is not a reason for avoiding buying a machine, but stresses the importance of making sure that the machine you buy is able to perform the tasks you require of it.

Here is an example to illustrate this process. Dr Green works in a small hospital which does not yet have an internal network. She wishes to purchase a machine for use at home. She wants to be able to use a word-processor to produce her research dissertation, do statistical analysis and also contact several friends, who live abroad, by electronic mail (e-mail). She feels it is unlikely that she will have to share word-processing files with other people.

Dr Green wants to be able to:

- Word-process in order to write, edit and print papers and letters.
- Carry out statistical tests for her dissertation.
- Prepare graphs for the dissertation.
- Prepare charts and slides for presentations.
- Send and receive e-mail.
- Print out the work which she produces.

Dr Green would be well advised to ensure that if at any time she does need to share word-processing, graphical or statistical files with colleagues that they use compatible products. Collaboration with local colleagues is probably best achieved by sharing documents on floppy disk (but see section below: Computer viruses). Adding a modem to her PC will enable her to send and receive messages and documents electronically. Her friends can be contacted via e-mail and to achieve this she will need to fit an internal (fitted within the computer – cheaper) or external (sits outside the computer and can therefore be carried between machines if needed) modem. She will also need access to a telephone line, and will need to sign up with an Internet Service Provider (ISP) to allow her to send and receive e-mails. This will also offer her access to the

---

* Software: computer programs are known as software. It is the software which determines what tasks a computer performs.

† Hardware: the physical components of a computer. It is the hardware which determines the limits within which a computer performs its tasks. For example, a computer without a CD-ROM drive will not read CD-ROM disks, regardless of which software is running.

World Wide Web (WWW). Dr Green will also need to buy a printer. Printers can use black or white or colour and work at various speeds from 1.5 to 16 or more pages a minute. Dr Green therefore needs to balance her needs with her budget. For most practical work such as writing a dissertation, a black and white printer which produces 4 or more pages a minute will be more than acceptable quality (see glossary definitions of laser, LED, ink-jet and dot matrix printers).

RESEARCH TASKS WHICH CAN BE ASSISTED BY THE USE OF A COMPUTER

In order to see how using a computer can help in research, it is useful to look at the tasks and processes involved in research.

1. Data manipulation

The majority of data manipulation in research falls into three areas: word processing, numerical processing and statistical testing.

a. Word-processing

Word-processing programs allow an author to create and alter text much more easily than handwriting or typing. The word-processing programs listed in Table 9.2 are widely available, simple to use and are often available at considerable discount to members of staff and students of educational establishments. All popular word-processor programs have a facility to check your text for spelling, grammatical or typing errors, but be aware that a check on spelling will not find cases where the error is a valid, but inappropriate, word. For example, '*chick*' and '*chuck*' are 'valid' misspellings of *check*. Medicine as a discipline has an enormous vocabulary – it is said (possibly apocryphally) that a student of medicine learns more new words in the first year of study than a student of Russian. Not surprisingly, most of these words are not known to the spell-check software and will be flagged as errors. Fortunately, most word-processors will allow you to add these and other new words to the built-in dictionary. You will need to make sure that the UK version of the spell-checker has been selected otherwise American spelling alternatives will be provided.

Most word-processing programs will also allow you to insert tables and pictures (either drawings or digital photographs) in the text. If you are interested in producing a newsletter or magazine-style articles, *Desktop Publishing Programs* (DTPs) allow you much more control of how columns of text behave on the page. If you look at a newspaper, you will notice that stories may finish in the middle of a page and continue several pages later. This sort of control over text flow is not possible in a standard word-processing package.

Table 9.2 *Common software processing packages. Most of these are available for Windows and Macintosh computers*

Package type	Program	Manufacturer
Word-processing	Word	Microsoft Ltd
	WordPerfect	Corel Ltd
	Lotus WordPro	Lotus Development Corporation
Spreadsheet (to hold and manipulate data)	Excel	Microsoft Ltd
	Quattro Pro	Corel Ltd
	Lotus 1–2–3	Lotus Development Corporation
Drawing packages (object based)	Corel DRAW!	Corel Ltd
	MicroGrafix Draw	MicroGrafix
	Adobe Illustrator	Adobe Ltd
Paint packages (pixel based to allow images/ photographs to be altered)	Corel Photopaint	Corel Ltd
	Adobe Photoshop	Adobe Ltd
	Paint Shop Pro	JASC In.
Presentation graphics	PowerPoint	Microsoft Ltd
	Corel Presents!	Corel Ltd
	Freelance	Lotus Development Corporation
	Harvard Graphics	Software Publishing Corporation
Databases (to hold and manipulate data)	Access	Microsoft Ltd
	Visual dBase	Borland Ltd
	Claris Filemaker Pro	Claris
	IdeaList	Blackwell Scientific Publications
	Visual FoxPro	Microsoft

b. Numerical processing

A spreadsheet looks like a sheet of children's squared paper – but the squares (cells) are active. You can type in numerical data or mathematical formulae expressing the relationships between the cells and numbers. For example, examine Table 9.3, a small spreadsheet. It contains data (heights and weights) which are entered as numbers. The column headed BMI (body mass index), although it displays as numbers, actually contains a hidden formula which expresses the relationship between BMI, height and weight. Entering the new data causes the BMI figure to update instantly. Most spreadsheet packages will perform a wide variety of basic statistical packages, but most lack the most esoteric functions used in medical research. Fully featured statistical packages are available for the PC, but tend to be expensive as they have relatively restricted markets.

Table 9.3 *Example spreadsheet*

Patient	Height	Weight	BMI
1	1.72	89	30.1
2	1.56	78	32.1
3	1.54	65	27.4
4	1.65	70	25.7
5	1.77	76	24.3
6	1.48	76	34.7
Mean	1.62	75.7	29.0

c. Statistical tests

The modern computer has revolutionized statistical analysis. It is now possible to perform in minutes analyses which only a few years ago required access to large mainframe computers. Simpler calculations, such as means and standard errors can now be done almost instantaneously and you will be able to perform them with minimal effort. There are potential drawbacks to this approach:

- There is a great temptation to proceed without the advice of a qualified statistician or to perform a wide variety of statistical procedures until one generates a favourable result.
- Although statistical programs will generate numerical results quickly, they offer little or no advice about interpretation. You need to know why you have done each test and the relevance of each positive and negative result.
- A common pitfall is to analyse a large number of variables and discover that one is 'significant' at, say, the 5% level. A moments thought will reveal that if you test 100 variables you should expect about 5 to show 'significant' deviation from the expected at this level of probability.
- Finally, since it is possible to reanalyse data as each new observation becomes available, there is again a temptation to stop analysing as soon as the results show 'significance'. These issues are addressed in greater detail in Chapters 6 to 8.

2. Data acquisition

A major step in any research project is the collection of data. This includes not only the experimental data, but also includes research protocols, references to prior published work and information culled from reference texts or databases. Input into the computer can be via a number of routes:

- Electronic, where the data are accepted in electronic format from another source (which may be another computer or a piece of specialized hardware such as a *scanner*). Textual information, including bibliographic material can be obtained and down-loaded from electronic databases such as MEDLINE or BIDS, or from pre-existing documents (see Chapter 4).

- Manual input where the data are typed into the computer by a human operator. Manual entry is most commonly used for entering written material or creating new drawings or diagrams. This is often time-consuming. Voice-recognition software is improving in performance and may become the primary route for data entry in future years.
- In some specialities, direct transmission from other equipment such as laboratory analysers is commonly used.

3. Data storage

Formal storage of data is performed by a group of programs known as *databases*. Three basic forms exist: flat-file, relational and free text databases. All allow you to store information, to sort it and to select data matching a given set of criteria – for example all patients with a given post code.

- Flat-file databases behave like electronic versions of the familiar card index. Each entry in the database (called a 'record') is complete in itself and does not refer to any other. All the records have the same structure, so it is not generally possible to store, for example, both bibliographic references and experimental data in the same database. Flat-file databases are easy to set up and use, but are restricted in their versatility. They also have problems with maintenance. Consider a laboratory ordering system based around a flat-file database. Table 9.4 shows a small section of the stock. If LabBits Inc. moves offices, the many independent entries in the database will have to be updated. This problem can be avoided by the use of a relational database.

Table 9.4 *Flat-file stock system*

Reagent	Supplier Name	Invoice Address	Phone Number
Sodium bromide	LabBits Inc.	123 Clements Road, Hull	796 87987
Sodium chloride	LabBits Inc.	123 Clements Road, Hull	796 87987
Sodium fluoride	Fluorides'R'Us	222 Halogen Way, Humberside	656 7687
Sodium iodide	LabBits Inc.	123 Clements Road, Hull	796 87987

- In a relational database, different types of information are in separate areas called tables and can be related to each other in a logical manner. Tables 9.5 and 9.6 show two sections of the same laboratory ordering system based around a relational database. If LabBits Inc. moves offices now, only the entry in the 'Suppliers' table needs to be changed.

Table 9.5 *Relational stock control system*

Reagent	Supplier code
Sodium bromide	L0010
Sodium chloride	L0010
Sodium fluoride	F4544
Sodium iodide	L0010

Table 9.6 *Relational stock control system*

Supplier code	Supplier Name	Invoice Address	Phone Number
L0010	LabBits Inc.	123 Clements Road, Hull	796 87987
G5655	General Equipment Co.	General House, Halifax	434 3213
F4544	Fluorides'R'Us	222 Halogen Way, Humberside	656 7687

- Neither of these forms of database performs well with data that are very variable in size and layout, such as bibliographic references or other large quantities of textual information. For these purposes, free-text databases have also been developed. These are more versatile than flat-file or relational databases, but are much slower at manipulating their data.

4. Data presentation

All research aims to communicate new information to others. Many different methods of presentation and channels of communication are available.

a. E-mail

Electronic mail represents a quick, convenient and cheap method of communicating with co-workers and of sharing information. At present, permanent e-mail access to the Internet is more commonly available to staff and students at academic institutions than those working within hospitals as hospital networks are commonly kept isolated from the outside world for reasons of security. This isolation is breaking down, and the creation of the NHS Network will speed this process.

- In order to access the Internet you will need a local network with Internet connection or you can purchase access through an Internet Service Provider (ISP) to which you connect via a standard telephone line.
- E-mails typically arrive at their destination within a few minutes of transmission wherever the destination in the world. E-mail is usually composed of plain text messages, but fully formatted word-processor

documents, pictures or other computer files can be sent 'attached' to an e-mail (as a file attachment).

b. Presentation graphics

Computers allow a range of presentation formats to be created:

- It is now common practice to prepare overhead transparency foils or projection slides on computer. Most laser or ink-jet printers can directly print overhead transparency sheets.
- It is also possible to project the computer output directly onto the projector screen using either a video-projector or OHP platen – an LCD device which connects to the computer and sits on the OHP allowing the contents of the computer screen to be projected onto the projector screen. Both these devices have a reduced image quality; however, they offer the ability to add animation and interaction to the presentation.
- Most modern presentation packages support the inclusion of digital video that allows communication of information which may be hard or impossible to convey using static images.

c. Diagram and graph drawing

Nearly all word-processing and spreadsheet packages include basic drawing tools that are adequate for simple illustrations. Computer drawing packages fall into two categories: *pixel-based* and *object-based*:

- A pixel-based drawing package treats the image as a series of coloured dots. This is the format which scanners and digital cameras produce. Pixel-based images suffer from two drawbacks. First, attempts to scale them often produce ugly results with jagged edges. Figure 9.1 shows a pixel-based image of a diagonal line before and after magnification.
- Another drawback to pixel-based drawing packages is that they are less easy to edit. Moving a section of a pixel-based image leaves an ugly hole which must be tediously redrawn. The paint-packages that come with most new systems are all pixel-based editors.

Figure 9.1 *A bitmap line magnified*

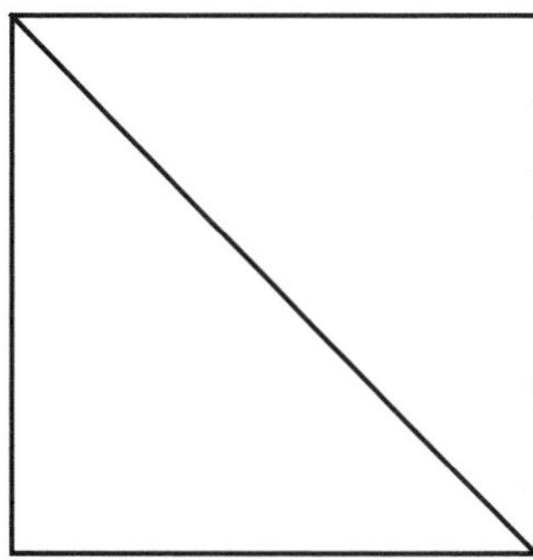

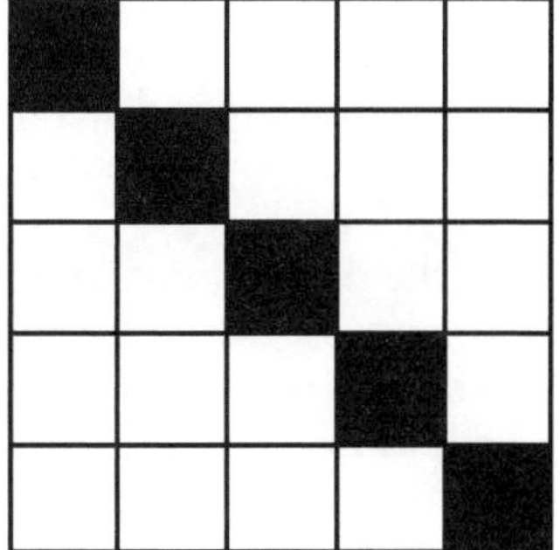

- In an object-based drawing package, all elements of a diagram are stored within the computer as electronic descriptions: the line-in-a-box seen in Figure 9.1 might be stored as 'Box: position 0,0 5 cm by 5 cm. Line: position 1,1 length 3 angle 45'. As a result, if it becomes necessary to edit the line or the box, only that specific part is altered. The other picture components are unaffected. This is very useful when the layout of a diagram needs to be altered to fit on a page.

TYPES OF PERSONAL COMPUTERS (PCs)

Most desktop PCs fall into one of two camps – the 'PC compatible' (most manufacturers) and the Macintosh (made by Apple Computers). Software written for one machine will not normally run on the other and moving data between systems can prove difficult. How do you choose which to use?

- Think about what you need to do with your PC. If you need to share data with a group of Macintosh users, or you must run a piece of software that is only available for the Macintosh, then you must buy a Macintosh.
- If most of your colleagues use PCs running MSDOS or Windows and you wish to share files, then you will probably be better off with a PC-compatible.

COMPUTER VIRUSES AND OTHER MALICIOUS SOFTWARE

Every few months, the papers announce that on some date a computer virus is going to wreak havoc with the nation's computer systems. Unfortunately, they never tell you what you should do about it. Some viruses are relatively harmless, some more dangerous.

If you want to protect yourself from loss of data, you should ask yourself some simple questions:

- Is my computer at risk from infection? (The answer is 'yes' if you ever receive disks from colleagues, bring disks in from your home PC, use magazine cover disks (including CDs), install commercial software or if your PC is connected to the Internet). In almost all cases the answer, therefore, is 'yes'!
- Is the data on my computer valuable? Valuable does not mean simply financial value. Writing documents and dealing with your research findings represents a large investment in your own time as well as any additional costs such as purchasing statistical help, etc. If your PC contains current research or other data that would be difficult to replace, you should also consider that valuable.

- Is my machine currently adequately protected? The answer is only 'yes' if you have installed a working copy of a reliable anti-virus (AV) software package, that the package is up-to-date (several new viruses are created each week) and that it is used – software which lies dormant on the hard drive does not protect your system.

What is a computer virus?

A virus is simply a program written to have special capabilities. As an absolute minimum, a computer virus can copy itself into other programs – in biological terms it 'infects' them. A well written virus leaves your computer working just as you would expect – it's only while you are using your PC that the virus can copy itself.

Where do they come from?

Programmers write computer viruses. They do not spontaneously generate themselves. Knowingly spreading them is now a criminal offence in many countries (including the UK).

Why do programmers write them?

Because they can? It's an interesting field for psychological investigation but there are no simple answers. Why do people vandalize bus shelters or spray graffiti?

How do they spread?

Viruses travel mainly in programs. Two sorts are common:

- 'File' viruses that infect program files. File viruses travel from machine to machine on floppy disk or via networks.
- 'Boot sector' viruses which infect a special area of a disk which 'boots' and starts up the computer when you turn it on. Boot sector viruses travel only via floppy disk.

What can a virus do?

A computer virus can do anything any other program can do. It may do something relatively harmless, such as play a tune. Some viruses tamper with your word-processing documents and insert insulting comments! More sinister viruses delete files or even wipe the computer's hard drive completely clean. Potentially most damaging in commercial circles are viruses that subtly alter data – add a few digits here, exchange a few there. If the accounts of a business are attacked by this sort of virus, by the time they realize what's going on, it may be too late.

What can't a virus do?

It can't do anything a program can't do. It can't do physical damage. It can't spread to another computer unless a network or modem connects the computers, or unless you take an infected floppy disk from one machine to the other.

Should I be worried?

Unfortunately, universities and other research centres are prime sites for the spread of computer viruses. If you value your work, you should take steps to protect it.

How do I protect my data?

- Firstly, *keep copies*. That way, you're unlikely to lose more than one copy.
- Secondly, use reliable anti-virus software.
- Thirdly, develop a suspicious mind.

You mentioned other malicious software – like what?

It is possible to write a program which does something unpleasant (like delete all your data), name it NICEGAME.EXE and make it available in a web-site or upload it to a 'bulletin board' from where people may copy it. It may even play a nice game, but delete files once in a while. Such a program is called a 'Trojan', after the 'Trojan Horse' of Greek legend. Only use software from reliable sources and you shouldn't have any problems.

How do anti-virus programs work?

Two basic techniques are used:

- Looking for known viruses.
- Looking for changes in existing files.

All the major anti-virus software vendors have enormous libraries of viruses. These known viruses are used to generate fingerprinting techniques that look at programs on disk to see if they contain a known virus. This technique will not find a new virus (until the company devise and issue a new fingerprint list, which most do monthly or quarterly). New viruses can also be detected by the changes they make to the files they infect.

Dealing with virus infection

Don't panic. Computer viruses are not like smallpox – they will not spread while you stop and think. Most AV software is capable of repairing most infected files – although it cannot bring back most deleted or destroyed files. Dealing with a virus outbreak is tedious, but not difficult. The basic steps are laid out below, but if you're at all unsure contact your PC support to discuss things before trying any heroics.

First, confirm that there is a genuine virus problem by using an up-to-date anti-virus program.

- Follow the instructions in your AV software manual to remove infected files from the PC. Re-scan the PC to make sure the viruses have been eradicated successfully.
- Get a highlighter pen.
- Gather together all your floppy disks. If you share a PC at home or in the office, get everyone to collect all their disks. Bring them to a PC.

For each floppy disk in turn:

- Make sure that the write-protect tab is slid to close the protect hole.
- Use your AV software to scan and confirm each disk is clean or remove the virus from the disk if it is infected.
- If it reports the disk is free of viruses, remove it from the drive, mark the disk label with the highlighter. The purpose of using the highlighter is that the chances are fairly good that you missed a few disks – in lockers, desks, jackets etc. Over the next few months, if you come across a disk which is not highlighted, you will know it has not been scanned and should be regarded as suspect,

If you cannot disinfect the disk, the best thing to do is reformat it. Put it on one side for now. Once you have scanned all your disks, format the unsalvageable disks using the 'unconditional format' option, and then re-scan them and mark them with the highlighter.

DATA SECURITY

One important feature of all forms of electronic data is that it is much simpler to copy and share than data stored physically. In addition, electronic copies do not degrade with each generation of copying – they are perfect copies of the original. A copied photographic slide is usually of noticeably lower quality than the original and may appear 'washed out'. Third and fourth generation photocopied documents may be difficult to read, but a hundredth generation digital copy is identical to the original in every way. Data in files can be changed rapidly and reliably using the computer. This changeability of data is the computer's great strength – but it is also a potential weakness. It is difficult to lose five papers, three graphs, and 12 pages of experimental results if they are all paper documents, but if they are all files on the same floppy disk, they can be lost or damaged much more easily.

Having multiple copies of your work is a vital safeguard. Computers do fail – they are also a frequent target for thieves. Disks get lost and damaged and occasionally you may want to refer back to an old draft of a paper. Make frequent *back-up* copies (for day-to-day security) and keep *archives* of old versions. You can protect yourself from potential loss of data by looking after your information is a sensible way. It is not difficult – here are some disaster scenarios and simple suggestions to make sure they don't happen to you.

Disk problems?

- Disks are physical objects, and like any physical object they can be damaged, lost or stolen. Don't have only one copy of your important files. Keep copies. Ideally, keep copies of any current work on your main home or office machine and on floppy disk. That way you can still work on a project if you leave the disk at home one day. It's also a good idea to label your disks. Each disk comes with a sticky label. Remove old labels before applying new ones or they tend to curl up inside the disk drive!
- You may receive the message 'General Failure reading disk in drive A:' when trying to access a file. This is usually due to physical damage to your disk. Disks have a long life but it is not infinite, and they are surprisingly delicate if mistreated. It is possible to copy disks, and all the files on them but obviously you have to do this before the disk gets damaged. Use good quality disks from a reliable manufacturer.
- Don't put disks in your pocket. If dust, grit, or fluff get inside the disk, they can scratch the delicate surface. Unlike paper copies, where spilling ink on one page leaves the others legible, a small area of damage to a disk can leave the whole thing unreadable. Keep disks clean. An envelope or small plastic bag is fine. Most large stationers sell 'disk mailers'. These are small semi-rigid plastic boxes that will hold and protect two floppy disks.
- Don't get disks wet, and don't keep them under a telephone or beside your loudspeakers. Keep them away from magnets. If you have an electronic pocket organizer with an alarm facility, keep it away from your disks. Keep it away from your credit cards too – the magnetic strip can get corrupted. Another commonly carried item that can create a strong (and potentially damaging) magnetic field is the mobile phone.

How to recover from unintentional errors

Physical loss and wear and tear are important threats to your data, but the biggest threat is human error. It is easy in a moment's inattention to delete the wrong file, or save a two-line note using the same name as your 50-page paper. The best defence against this sort of problem is organization. Some ideas to overcome this are:

- Name your files sensibly: don't call every paper you write 'PAPER.DOC' Devise some sensible naming system that you can remember.
- Keep different versions of important files: move on to a new version number when you feel you have done a 'reasonable' amount of work (i.e. an amount you wouldn't want to lose!). Don't get too carried away – there's no point doing 10 minutes file copying to secure five minutes typing.
- Keep copies: make backups of your important files and keep them at a different site from the main computer.

Backing up your data

Looking after the security of your work is vitally important. Fortunately, it is also simple. There are two important concepts – *backups* and *archives*.

What is a backup?

- A backup is simply a copy of all your files which is not held on your computer.
- If you copy the files to another disk or computer and keep that disk away from your computer (at home, if you do most work at work, or at work, if you do most work at home) then you will be safe from most disasters such as fires.

The simplest technique is to label *three* sets of disks (or tapes, see later) with sufficient capacity on each to hold all your data. At regular intervals, copy all your current work on to one set of disks. Next time, use the second set, and then the third. After that, go back to the first set of disks and cycle round them again. The rotation of disks allows you a 'lag-time' to discover any loss of data or file damage.

How frequently should I backup?

The purpose of backup is to save your data and time. If you don't mind re-doing a week's work, then weekly backups will suffice. During busy periods you may prefer to make a backup every day or few days. It is a personal balance between the time committed to doing the backup, and the amount of work that would have to be redone if your data become lost.

What is an archive?

Using the backup strategy mentioned above, all copies of the data (on the computer and on the three sets of disks) are relatively recent. Occasionally, you may want to refer back to an older draft; perhaps to restore some writing you had removed. An archive is a set of backups which is not recycled, but is simply kept safely in case it is needed.

Archives are generally made much less frequently than backups – perhaps monthly or quarterly.

How do I make a backup?

This depends on the amount of data involved. Small quantities, such as would fit on one or two floppy disks, require no special extra purchases. Larger quantities of data may require many disks, and some data files may grow so large that they will not fit on a single disk. At this point it is worth considering specialized backup hardware solutions, such as a *tape streamer*. Bear in mind that if you are working on an institutional network, there may well be a centralized backup device. Contact your IT unit and enquire. Small tape streamers suitable for domestic or small office use can be purchased for as little as £100 and come with software which simplifies the backup process.

PROTECTING YOURSELF

You may have heard about health and safety issues relating to the use of computers. Although most problems are less likely in people using computers for only limited lengths of time, it's only sensible to be aware of potential problems that you can avoid easily.

1. Repetitive strain injury (RSI)

RSI is collective term for a group of musculoskeletal problems which seem to share a common causation – the repeated performance of small movements for long periods of time. RSI is less common in people who have been taught a 'good typing style' than in the self-taught 'hunt and peck' typist. Typing tutor programs are widely available and not expensive. Try to spend a few minutes a day practising. You may feel that you are too busy, but the improvement in your typing speed and skills will soon save you time – and you'll be acquiring a skill which will protect you from injury and which you will use for the rest of your life.

2. Sitting posture

The position at which you work is also important in preventing back, neck, and shoulder problems. Many of these problems can be avoided by adjusting the setting of the computer.

Figure 9.2 illustrates the important points. Note:

- Eyes level with top of screen.
- Elbows level with desk.

Figure 9.2 *An effective sitting position*

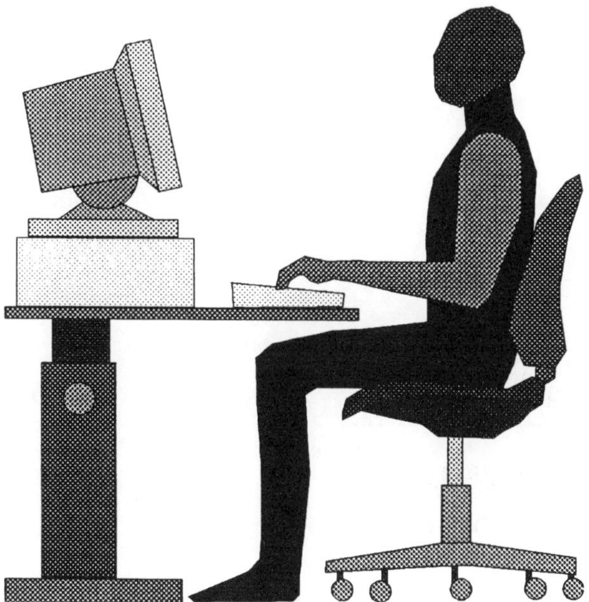

- Wrist held above keyboard, so the wrist is *flexed* not *extended.*
- Hips level with knees.
- Feet flat on floor.
- Get the chair/desk height matched, and then raise the monitor if necessary.

3. Eyestrain

This is a relatively common complaint. To avoid eyestrain, set the monitor height as described above. Try to avoid reflections from windows or room lights. Every 10 minutes or so, stop working for a moment and stare at the wall, out of the window, or generally into the distance. Try to avoid siting your computer in an area lit by fluorescent lighting.

By doing these very basic things, you will be able to use your computer in helpful ways. Ways which increase your efficiency and ability to complete tasks and at the same time to do this without causing any long-term physical problems to yourself.

KEY POINTS

- The personal computer (PC) offers an affordable and highly effective tool for research.
- Buy the right computer and software to carry out the tasks you require.
- Get to know how to use the software you need effectively.
- Beware of computer viruses. Invest in anti-virus software with regular updates and make sure you have a routine way of backing up your files.
- Make sure that you have a good posture, lighting and working environment while working at your computer.
- Talk to the experts, they will help you choose what you need.

ADDITIONAL READING

Lee, N., Millman, A. ABC of medical computing: choosing a computer system. *British Medical Journal,* 1995; **311,** 46–9.

Lee, N., Millman, A. ABC of medical computing: CD ROM's, multimedia and optical storage systems. *British Medical Journal,* 1995; 311, 675–8.

Lee, N., Millman, A. ABC of medical computing: linking your computer to the outside world. *British Medical Journal,* 1995; 311, 381–4.

Lee, N., Millman, A. ABC of medical computing: storing and managing data on a computer. *British Medical Journal,* 1995; 311, 562–5.

GLOSSARY

CD-ROM (Compact disk read-only memory): a large capacity, cheap store medium. A single CD-ROM disk can hold the equivalent of roughly 400 floppy disks, but once made cannot be edited. Commonly used for distributing programs.

Digital camera: a hand-held device which captures images directly in digital format. Digital cameras are becoming cheaper and widely available. Professional models are expensive and their use is therefore restricted to projects with very special requirements.

Dot-matrix printer: a printer which makes marks on paper by hitting an ink-impregnated ribbon with small pins. The resulting characters are made up of a matrix of dots large enough to be visible, hence the name. Dot-matrix printers are slow, noisy and of low print quality. Some models can print colour. They can print multi-part (self-carbon) stationery and can take continuous stationery. Often used to print labels or invoices. Not recommended for general office use.

Ink-jet printer: a printer which makes marks on paper by squirting small dots of ink on to the paper. The resulting characters are made up of a matrix of dots usually too small to be visible as dots. Ink-jet printers are slower than laser printers, but almost silent in operation and of reasonable print quality. Some models can print colour. They are commonly used as home printers and are the cheapest method of colour printing and are often used to print overheads on a special type of transparency. The ink is often not waterproof and their use for address labels may therefore not be appropriate.

Internet: a 'network of networks' – an extended international network which allows rapid communication across the globe. It is essentially unregulated and exists by the mutual cooperation of the companies and institutions which own the components.

Laptop computer: see notebook computer

Laser printer: these are now the commonest form of printers seen in office use. They mark the paper by a process similar to that seen in photocopiers. A charged drum is scanned by the laser. Toner (a fine black powder) adheres to the charged areas of the drum and then is transferred to the paper. The paper is then heated and the toner fuses to the paper. Laser printers are very quiet in use and produce high quality text and graphics. They can print on paper or appropriate overhead transparency foils. Normal foils and some forms of special letter headings may melt in the printer and should not be used. Most laser printers print only in black and white. Colour models are available, but are expensive. Laser printers are a type of page printer. Page printers form an electronic image of the page in their internal memory and then print the entire page at once. They are quick for printing text, and very quick at producing second and subsequent pages of text or graphics.

LED printer: close relative of the laser printer. Instead of a laser scanning the charged drum, a series of close-packed light-emitting diodes is used. Apart from that the functioning of the devices is identical. See Laser printer.

Modem: a device which allows information from computers to be converted into tones which can pass along standard telephone lines. The modem encodes the digital information by *mo*dulating a carrier tone. A complementary modem connected to the receiving computer *dem*odulates the tones to retrieve the information, hence modem.

Mouse: an input device that allows a pointer to be moved around the screen and choices made (e.g. buttons clicked).

Multimedia computers: computers which have been fitted with a sound-card, speakers and a CD-ROM. Allows games, video and interactive materials to be used. Typically use moving images and sound to convey information. Advantageous to use a larger monitor (15 inches (38 cm) or larger) if purchasing this option.

Network: a system of connecting computers so that they can share information and resources, such as secure storage or expensive printers. Small offices can set up a network for their own use for less than £30 per computer. Larger networks have greater overheads, both in the equipment needed to support them, and the work involved in administering the network.

Notebook computer: a computer which has been designed to be small and self-contained, but which is still capable of operating standard software. To make a computer self-contained, many design compromises have to be made. A traditional glass-tube monitor is too large and bulky, so notebooks use liquid crystal displays. Originally, these were monochrome, but colour displays are becoming less expensive. To keep the size down, the keyboard layout is reduced and many keys take on more than one function. This can cause problems for touch-typists. In addition, the internal arrangement of components is usually proprietary to each manufacturer. As a result, notebook computers are much more expensive than the equivalent desktop computer and expensive or impossible to upgrade.

Printer: device for creating printed copies of electronic documents. A number of types exist, each with advantages and disadvantages. It is often possible to share a printer between users via a network or electronic switch if the machines are close enough together. See Dot-matrix printer, Ink-jet printer, Laser printer.

Scanner: a desk-top device, usually slightly larger than an A4 page, which takes a physical image and converts it into an electronic format. Scanners may be capable of producing black and white or colour images (more expensive). Connecting to the computer may be via a dedicated interface card which fits internally (and hence prevents use with a notebook, or moving the scanner between computers) or via the printer connection, although this may cause problems if you wish to use your printer while the scanner is attached.

Tape streamer: a specialized piece of hardware which allows large quantities of data to be copied to tape cartridges for storage (e.g. to backup the entire hard drive).

Word processor: a piece of computer software which simplifies the editing of text. Most word processors allow the insertion of table, graphs, diagrams and pictures. Once created, a word processor document can be printed or transmitted electronically.

World Wide Web (WWW or W^3): one of the information services provided on the Internet. The WWW is based around a method of describing documents which does not depend on any specific form of computer or display. As a result, although Web pages are less versatile then might be wished, they permit the easy sharing of data between users. Within medicine, the WWW is most useful as a source of information (many databases can now be searched via the WWW) and of educational material.

Chapter Ten

Maintaining momentum

Anne Worrall-Davies

INTRODUCTION

Maintaining momentum can be one of the most difficult tasks in doing research. Even the most dedicated and enthusiastic researchers get 'stuck' or lose motivation at some stage, particularly in a larger research project. Losing momentum can occur at any stage in a project and for a variety of reasons. The purpose of this chapter is to identify obstacles to research, and to create a useful framework for overcoming these obstacles.

WHY YOU LOSE MOMENTUM

In the survey of senior registrar trainees described in Chapter 2,[1] 50.9% had a research project that had failed or was stuck. In over 20% of projects where data had been collected, the study remained uncompleted because of problems with data analysis or writing up the study. The causes vary depending on whatever stage you lose momentum and can be divided into internal or external factors (Table 10.1). This division is based on educational research looking at aspects of learning.

Internal factors are causes of loss of momentum located within yourself and can be divided into:

- A lack of knowledge and skills about the research topic or the process of research (e.g. research design, statistical tests, use of computers etc.).
- Negative attitudes towards your research.
- Previous adverse research experience.
- Personal belief systems about research.
- A lack of ability to prioritize time for research and assertively protect this.

External factors may be divided into:

- Practical issues (clinical commitments and work demands, availability of information technology etc. – see Chapter 2).

- Access to effective research supervision.
- The attitudes and support of peers, friends and family around you.

Table 10.1 *Checklist identifying blocks to your motivation*

Internal factors:		
1. Lack of knowledge/research skills.	Yes	No
2. Negative attitudes towards research/procrastination etc.	Yes	No
3. Previous adverse experiences in research.	Yes	No
4. Negative personal beliefs about research.	Yes	No
5. Research isn't a priority for me.	Yes	No
External factors:		
1. Lack of resources (access to computer, money, etc.).	Yes	No
2. Job demands make research difficult.	Yes	No
3. No access to an effective supervisor.	Yes	No
4. Negative view of research by your peers/colleagues.	Yes	No

OVERCOMING OBSTACLES TO RESEARCH: INTERNAL FACTORS

1. Lack of knowledge and research skills

Many trainees and clinicians feel that they ought to have gained the knowledge and skills to do research and many are very aware of their shortfall and lack of skills. This is often the case where computer skills are concerned. In the survey of all psychiatric trainees in Northern and Yorkshire Region described in Chapter 2, many trainees felt they lacked the skills to use new technology. Some clear sex differences were apparent with more female SRs believing they lack the skills needed to use a computer, (male 21.9%; female 48.0%; chi squared = 4.31, 1df, $P<0.037$), and to use a statistical package (chi squared 8.60, 1df, $P<0.033$). Whether this belief is a subjective feeling, or objectively accurate, it is clear that this perception is a major issue for many trainees. These beliefs may lead to losing momentum at the start of a project, and at any point in carrying out the project. Certain areas of the research process often disproportionately worry new researchers. These particularly include times when research design or statistical issues are highlighted. Table 10.2 summarizes a wide range of possible research skills you could aim to achieve.

The survey found that only 7% of trainees described their research training as 'good', with 52.6% describing their training as 'adequate'. Worryingly, 38.6% believed their training was 'poor' or 'non-existent'. It is worth remembering that while many trainees have gained some knowledge

Table 10.2 *Core research knowledge and skills (adapted from Owens et al.[2])*

You and your supervisor should be able to:

1. Pose a research question: turn general aims into specific hypotheses.
2. Conduct a competent computerized literature search.
3. Understand the principles of the key types of study design.
4. Know how to select populations, samples and control groups.
5. Understand how to deal with bias and confounding.
6. Understand the validity of scales, measures of agreement and principles of screening.
7. Calculate and use raw and category-specific rates of disease.
8. Calculate and use appropriately relative and attributable risk, odds ratios.
9. Appropriately describe data in text, tables, figures and charts.
10. Use and understand confidence intervals and simple hypothesis tests, type I and II errors.
11. Understand the principles of power calculations.
12. Collect data appropriately and enter in a computer database.
13. Analyse data appropriately using a computer statistics package.
14. Understand the nature and principles of systematic reviews and meta-analysis.

and skills in research, it is unlikely that they will possess a high knowledge base of how to put this into practice unless they have undergone additional practical research training or undertaken research themselves. As an analogy, you would never attempt to offer psychotherapy to a client after only reading a book on it. Instead you would first seek specific training and clinical supervision. The situation is the same with research. You should not feel despondent about not having all the core knowledge and skills you need – you will gain these by doing and being supervised in research, thereby discovering a range of practical problems and difficulties that must be overcome, and finding ways of achieving this.

Action plan

To avoid losing momentum due to a lack of the relevant knowledge and skills, first decide what you *need* to learn. Look through Table 10.2 in detail (preferably with your supervisor). You will not need to know or be adept in every area detailed there. Try to prioritize 'core' and 'optional' knowledge for the study you are doing. Discuss with your supervisor what skills you should prioritize as your main learning goal in the current study.

Having decided for yourself the range of skills which you need to seek, identify local or national courses or in-house training to address these needs specifically. Word-processing, statistics, research methodology and design courses are increasingly being run by Trust R&D departments. They are often available locally free of charge. Look out for adverts or circulars that mention them. Many Trusts and University Departments have 'Forthcoming Training Events' or specific Research Training notice boards. Seek them out and take up appropriate opportunities on offer. If you know that you have a particular need, ask if there are any courses which address this. If none exist at present, ask if it is possible for one to be offered – or organize one yourself with Trust support.

2. Negative attitudes about research

There is a recognized cycle of psychological mood swings during a research project,[3] moving through:

- Euphoria.
- Boredom.
- Loss of motivation.
- Frustration.

The longer the project lasts the more likely you are to lose motivation. Being bored with repetitive tasks such as data entry, collating questionnaires, etc. is common. Being frustrated at not being able to have time to explore side issues that arise along the way is also to be expected. One way of overcoming this is to make a note of areas you would like to explore so that this can become the focus of another future study if you wish. However academically brilliant you are, only hard work and application can get you through a project. This can sometimes be difficult to accept intellectually. 'Research work is just that – (work)' is a useful maxim to remember.[3] When you feel that you are fed up with research and find that it isn't interesting and challenging all the time, remember it often isn't!

Action plan

- Set a research plan with project milestones on a weekly or monthly basis.
- Check yourself against it regularly and encourage your supervisor also to check it.
- Plan your work schedule in order to sandwich interesting parts of the project round boring tasks on a daily or weekly basis.
- Make sure you attain a proper balance between the different aspects of your work (research, clinical, managerial, special interest) and home life.
- If you are involved in a large piece of research (such as an MD), prepare for the long haul. Allocate time when you are not doing work. Ensure that you protect time such as weekends and holidays. This will help you prevent burnout.
- Talk to your colleagues, friends and family about your research and about any blocks you are having. Seek their encouragement and support.
- Consider setting up a supportive forum for trainees and colleagues doing research.
- Talk your concerns through with your supervisor.

3. Previous adverse research experiences

Having a bad experience with previous attempts at research may have put you off research for the future. In the survey of trainees in Northern and Yorkshire Region, 51% of senior registrars had experienced a previous failed attempt at research. If you are someone in the same situation, it is important for you to know that you are not alone!

Look back to your previous experience of research. At which stage has the research failed or stopped? There are numerous stages within the research process where progress may be halted (Table 10.3).

Table 10.3 *Where does research fail?*

Protocol stage.	18%
Ethical approval.	4%
Data collection.	29%
Data analysis.	18%
Writing up.	25%
Unable to find a publisher.	7%

Source: Survey of SRs in Psychiatry.[1]

N = 28 SRs who identified that they had been involved in a previously failed piece of research. 1 missing response.

Try to learn from your past experiences so that you can avoid making the same mistakes again:

- What are the factors that increased your motivation at the time – how can you build this into your research again?
- What factors hindered it, slowed it down or ultimately damaged your ability to do the research. How could you plan things differently this time to overcome it?

There are numerous possible reasons for your previous research losing its momentum. This might include:

- An absent supervisor.
- An overly-critical supervisor.
- A project you were not intrinsically interested in.
- Too many other competing demands.

Action plan

You need to talk to someone you respect but can trust, perhaps a peer colleague or a trusted senior colleague who has done research and therefore will almost certainly know exactly how you feel. Discuss what happened previously and adopt a problem-solving approach to avoid it happening this time round. A step by step approach to doing this is outlined in Chapter 2.

4. Negative personal beliefs about research

You may simply not see yourself as a researcher: 'I'm a clinician' or 'I'm not bright enough' or 'I'm not interested in research, that's for academics', or even 'It's a waste of time'. Be aware of these beliefs and consider how they might affect your feelings and actions towards research. If you find that you aren't doing things that you really wish to do because of the views of others it is important to try and question why this is.

Action plan

Your need to discuss with your supervisor and/or colleagues:

- Why you are doing research.
- What your research skills are, what suits you to do this particular project.
- Review your career development and whether research is a necessary part of your own continuing professional development.

5. Prioritization of research time

This is linked with the above attitudes. If you are unhappy with the concept of yourself as a researcher, or have had a previous bad experience in previous research, you may find that you just never have enough time to get on with your research. A lack of time is one of the two most common causes of failed research. Clinical pressures are undoubtedly present for every researcher unless he or she is in a full-time research post. If you find that finding time to do research is a major problem, try to examine your own motivations in this. If you do not have time to carry out research, by definition you are spending that time on something else. This involves an element of conscious or subconscious choice. Consider the advantages and disadvantages for you of this in the short and long term. Are these decisions likely to be helpful or cause you problems? If the latter, how can you overcome it?

Action plan

- You should look carefully at your time management to see whether you actually do not have enough time or whether you are choosing not to make the time – a hard and soul-searching task.
- Discuss this issue with trusted others. Their support and encouragement can be very helpful.

Prioritizing research means that you have actively to make some decisions. It doesn't just happen:

- You need to be very selective about taking on new work. Are there any current things that you are doing which you do not need to do.
- Avoid taking on new things no matter how attractive they seem at the time. They will only cause you difficulties later.
- If you are involved in a number of research topics and the quantity of them is preventing you advancing the main project, consider withdrawing from some of the other projects. Focus on those that are most likely to produce quality (peer-reviewed) publications.

OVERCOMING OBSTACLES TO RESEARCH: EXTERNAL FACTORS

1. Practical issues

A number of practical obstacles may lead to a loss of momentum in carrying out your research:

- Difficulty using or gaining access to computer equipment, statistical or research advice.
- The project relies on external funding which does not materialize.
- Shortage of time.
- Intrinsic design problems within the project (such as unrealistic expectations of what is achievable within the time, a lack of support from other collaborators, patients recruitment rates lower than expected etc.).

2. Excessive job demands

Part of your job as a trainee psychiatrist is to gain skills in research as well as clinical management. The local training committee, the Royal College of Psychiatrists and your college tutor will all be able to support you if you experience consistent problems in obtaining your research time as a result of your job. In most cases, however, this can be accomplished simply by discussing it with your current consultant trainer. These issues are discussed in greater length within Chapter 2.

3. Access to effective research supervision

Finding a supervisor who is right for you can be difficult. If you are carrying out research which is registered with a university for a higher degree, you may be allocated one or you may choose one who subsequently proves not to be as helpful as you anticipated. Adequate supervision and training is central to effective research; however, in the SR survey, although 61.4% of senior registrars felt that they received adequate supervision and support from trainers, only 28.1% felt that this was 'good'.

Attributes of an effective supervisor

- Supervisors need all the knowledge, skills and attitudes outlined in the earlier part of this chapter, or must be willing to acquire these.
- They must be proactive in suggesting contacts or involving others who have the expertise they lack.
- They should be able to offer you at least 1 hour/month supervision time regularly.
- Preferably they will be engaged in research themselves at least in the broad area of your research topic.
- They should possess good interpersonal and facilitative skills and be able to offer constructive suggestions and not belittle you.
- Should know when to 'strongly encourage' you to continue the research at times when you need this!
- You may also need to train your supervisor, and suggest how he or she may best address your needs.

4. The views of colleagues, peers, family and friends

Peers are very important and without them you may find yourself overwhelmed by the emotions outlined under internal factors (boredom, frustration etc.).

- Lay persons (friends, spouses) are useful for providing the big picture on a thorny issue, or to identify whether a protocol/article is clearly written, understandable and jargon-free.
- An intelligent reader outside the field of research can often pinpoint key problem areas you have failed to identify because you are too closely involved in the material. Remember your supervisor may reach this stage too.
- Remember that friends and relatives may sometimes collude with you to reinforce your decision to 'give-up' on research. Your research may have implications for them (for example writing up your project during 'home' time). This may be especially relevant if you have young children at home. In these situations, open discussion about this issue may be helpful in order to examine your motivations and fears concerning the research. Negotiating a specific 'protected' time to work and times when you will not work may offer a helpful and practical solution to this situation. Considering your decision in detail by using a cost-benefit analysis such as that described in Chapter 2 may be useful.

KEY POINTS

- You need to address loss of momentum early on to avoid becoming irrevocably stuck and never finishing the project.
- Be proactive and seek to maintain your momentum.
- Anticipate difficult times (e.g. around exams, job interviews, changes of job etc.).
- Identify the causes of lost momentum using the framework outlined in the chapter.
- Create an action plan using the suggestions in the chapter. Make it specific to you and your own situation.
- Action plans can be used both proactively to avoid losing momentum, and reactively to overcome specific problems which do arise in order to help you move forward in the project.
- Don't give up on the project, remember that everyone loses momentum at some point in a project.
- Enjoy your research time. It can be challenging and interesting.

REFERENCES

1. Williams, C. J., Curran, S. Research by senior registrars in psychiatry. *Psychiatric Bulletin*, 1998; **22**, 102–4.
2. Owens, D., House, A., Worrall, A. Research by trainees. *Psychiatric Bulletin*, 1995; **19**, 337–40.
3. Phillips, E., Pugh, D. S. *How to get a PhD*. 2nd edn. 1994; Open University Press, Buckingham.

Chapter Eleven

Get it published!

David Yeomans

INTRODUCTION

To publish your work is to reach an end-point in the research process. When your paper is published in a journal, you have demonstrable evidence of your ideas and hard efforts. It is a considerable achievement which will enhance your curriculum vitae and career prospects. However, getting your research published cannot be taken for granted. The process of publishing your work starts with your initial choice of project. Consider whether your research is *possible, achievable* and ultimately *publishable.* You should also consider the requirements of journals and their referees even when you begin to plan your research. This will avoid wasting a great deal of your time. One of the best ways to learn how to publish research is to join an established research group and learn from a good supervisor. In this environment you will develop all the skills you need.

WHY DO I WANT TO PUBLISH RESEARCH?

You should be able to answer this question before you start. Research may be your chosen career, in this case you should certainly be thinking about joining an active research team as early as possible. It is not easy to move into research full-time later on in life, although it is possible. Having research skills and a proven publication record is a benefit to you even if you do not have a long-term plan to develop research as a central part of your working life. There is a proven link between having a publication on your curriculum vitae and a successful job interview.[1, 2] It is worth deciding how much time you can devote to research while managing the rest of your job and private life. Many doctors begin a research project but do not complete it. Some finish the data collection but fail to get their paper accepted by a journal or as a conference presentation. Undoubtedly most will have acquired some research skills along the way. If you want to publish you are going to need *motivation.*

You must really want to do it! One useful rule before even starting your research is to ask yourself (or others) '*is it potentially publishable?*' If not, do you still want to do it or can you modify it so that it is?

WHERE TO START?

As a trainee, you should have several opportunities to find out about how to write up your research for publication:

- Journal clubs can bring you into contact with published work of all sorts, and may also introduce reading and analytical skills. When you read articles by others, on your own or in journal clubs, use this as an opportunity to think about how and why articles are put together and structured as they are.
- Courses on how to write and publish are regularly advertised in the *British Medical Journal* and may be of interest to you.
- If you attend Royal College or other conferences you will be able to talk to researchers in your field of interest and discover how research can be presented as posters, talks and abstracts.
- Senior colleagues will have a variety of personal experiences of writing up research. Seek their advice and comments on early drafts.

PUBLISH ON MY OWN OR WITH OTHERS?

If you glance through any journal you will see papers with contributions from several authors working in collaboration. These authors may be members of a research team, or may be junior staff and their supervisors. Some papers have been written by people in different countries sharing their resources, and some projects include specialists in different areas such as epidemiology, statistics and public health. Single author reports are still common, but you may find collaborative work with others can help you set goals and allocate different parts of the write-up so that the workload is fairly shared. It is worth openly discussing and agreeing what each author expects at the outset to avoid disputes later (e.g. who will be the first author?).

WHO IS MY AUDIENCE?

It would be marvellous to publish your first project in a high profile international journal, but is your work more suited to a nationally published journal or one aiming at a specialized readership? In order to decide what type of journal to write for, ask yourself:

- Who will be interested in my findings?
- What professional groups do I want to read the paper? For example, if you have carried out research in a casualty department, the work could be applicable to a casualty audience, a general practice audience, a liaison psychiatry, general psychiatry or general medical/surgical audience.
- You may want to aim the work at trainees or trainers. What are their different requirements?

WHERE CAN I PUBLISH?

You can publish in journals, books and conference abstracts. You can also publish electronically on the Internet.[3] Other options include local departmental documents or governmental reports. Many small projects are published as letters. There is a hierarchy of publications dependent upon the level of expert scrutiny to which your work is exposed. Well-known, long-established journals with stringent peer review and editorial control are the most read and prestigious places to publish. These journals include:

- *The American Journal of Psychiatry.*
- *Archives of General Psychiatry.*
- *British Journal of Psychiatry.*
- *British Medical Journal.*
- *The Lancet.*
- *Nature.*
- *New England Journal of Medicine.*

There are also specialist publications in a range of fields such as *Addiction, The Journal of Family Therapy* and the *Health Service Journal*. Your literature searching will reveal other journals publishing in your area of work. Colleagues can offer advice too. In general, peer-reviewed journals are seen as being more prestigious than those journals which accept or commission articles for publication without this quality requirement. Journals always state whether their policy is to send articles out for peer review. Normally those journals which do this will ask for you to submit more than one copy of your final paper to allow this to occur. You should seek to publish your articles in journals that will be read by the audience that you wish and which are peer-reviewed if possible.

If you are uncertain whether a particular journal will be interested in your research, consider asking them before submitting it. An editor will usually provide rapid feedback concerning whether their publication would consider your work. It is worth giving them a telephone call to discuss your work. Useful telephone numbers are given in the summary box at the end of the chapter.

WHAT IS MY BRIEF?

A brief is a specification, a set of aims and targets for your written work. You can set your own brief by deciding who you are trying to reach (target audience) and writing for them. You must also angle your paper towards the journal you will be submitting it to. The journal will publish *instructions for authors* which will further guide you.

Scientific writing tends to conform to a limited style. Some journals expect you to write an impersonal piece in the third person using what is called the passive voice. An example of this style is 'The patients were allocated randomly to each of the three experimental groups'. Other journals permit a more personal and active approach. The sample sentence above could be written like this: 'We allocated patients randomly to each of the three experimental groups.'

Most editors will appreciate:

- Simple English.
- Good grammar.
- An appropriate 'style' for their journal.
- Accurate punctuation.
- A clear structure to your paper.

WHAT IS A JOURNAL STYLE?

Read your target journal. Imagine how your piece would look in the 'house' style. You can find the detailed requirements about journal style in the *instructions for authors*. These may be published periodically (often in the first issue of the year), but every journal will draw your attention to the relevant edition which contains the instructions. These instructions may fill several pages. You must read them carefully. You will find advice about how to lay out your work. This can be very specific and include information on:

- Line spacing.
- Margin size.
- Page numbering.
- Headings (e.g. Introduction; Aims; Methods; Analysis; Results; Discussion).
- Number and style of tables, diagrams or pictures.
- The style and length of abstract.
- How to record authorship (important for blind peer-reviewing).

You may also be asked to provide multiple copies in writing and on computer disk in a variety of word-processing formats.

As well as formatting what you are writing into the correct journal style, you also need to ensure that the content of what you send is appropriate for the journal. What does your target journal expect you to say about ethics committee approval, or permission from patients to use clinical material? What sort of data analysis does the journal require. You must find this out and incorporate what you find into the writing process.

HOW DO I STRUCTURE MY REFERENCES?

Journals vary in the format of referencing that they use. Most use either the Harvard or Vancouver style.

Psychiatric Bulletin and the *British Journal of Psychiatry* use the Harvard style. The following is an example of a sentence written using this style of referencing:

Harvard style

This is similar to findings in other areas of psychotherapeutic research in which a linear relationship has been found between the logarithm of the number of sessions and the normalised probability of patient improvement (Howard *et al.,* 1993). Reported in (Treasure *et al.,* 1996).

Journal Article Reference: Harvard style:

TREASURE, J.L., TROOP, N.A. and WARD, A. (1996) An approach to planning services for bulimia nervosa. *British Journal of Psychiatry.* **169**, 551–554.

Book Chapter Reference: Harvard style:

HOWARD, K.L., ORLINSKY, D.E. and LUEGER, R.J. (1993) The design of clinically relevant outcome research: some considerations and an example. In *Research Foundations for Psychotherapy Practice* (eds M. Aveline and D Shapiro), pp. 215–231. Chichester: Wiley.

In contrast, the Vancouver style for the same sentence would be:

Vancouver style

This is similar to findings in other areas of psychotherapeutic research in which a linear relationship has been found between the logarithm of the number of sessions and the normalised probability of patient improvement.[1] Reported by Treasure.[2]

Book Chapter Reference: Vancouver style:

[1] Howard KL, Orlinsky DE, Lueger RJ. The design of clinically relevant outcome research: some considerations and an example. In: Aveline M, Shapiro D. ed. *Research Foundations for Psychotherapy Practice.* Chichester: Wiley, 1993: 215–231.

Journal Article Reference: Vancouver style:

[2] Treasure JL, Troop NA, Ward A. An approach to planning services for bulimia nervosa. *Br J Psych* 1996; **169**: 551–554.

HOW DO I PREPARE THE WORK FOR SUBMISSION?

You (and your colleagues) have set up the project, collected data, analysed it and developed your own conclusions. You have probably already used a word processor, statistical package, spreadsheet or database at least as part of the initial research. You have decided on your brief, target audience and favoured journal. You have the instructions for authors. All you have to do is write the final draft.

- Don't start writing yet! Think before you write.
- Ask yourself, 'What is the key message of the study?' Focus all that you write around this.
- Write out a plan so that you can impose a structure on what you write. Attempt to tell the story of why you did this research and what you found.

Table 11.1 summarizes the key elements required in order to impose a structure on what you write.

Table 11.1 *Imposing a structure on what you write*

1. *Tell the readers the rationale behind why you decided to do what you did.*
   This might include a brief background literature review stating what has been found before in this research area, what are the main questions that are unanswered and need to be addressed, the pitfalls in previous research – hence the reason for you doing this research.
2. *Tell the readers what you did.*
   The methods and practical aspects of your study, its data analysis and results.
3. *Tell them about the meaning and relevance of your results.*
   The discussion should cover the importance of the results, implications for practice, the limitations of the findings and the relative strengths and weaknesses of the experimental design and how the study was carried out.

Modify this basic structure to fit the style and content required by your target journal.

Writing a paper takes longer than you imagine. Once you have written a first draft:

- Leave for a while and come back to it.
- Revise and re-revise it.
- If you have written a very long paper, consider setting yourself a target to reduce the length by a third. You may well be asked to do this anyway by the prospective journal. Set yourself a target number of words (often specified in the *instructions to authors*).
- Ruthlessly cut out material that is irrelevant to the central message of the paper no matter how interesting it is to you. Save it for another paper.

- Read it with a critical eye and check for mistakes and discrepancies.
- Imagine you are a reviewer. What is the English like? Do the figures add up? Are the conclusions justified?

Once you are satisfied, show it to someone else for their constructive comments. It can help sometimes to be specific about what sorts of feedback you are wanting. Ask for comments about:

- What is good about the paper?
- Is the central message clear?
- What are the weaker areas of the paper?
- Ask for comments on each main section of the paper (Introduction, methods etc.).
- Ask for specific suggestions about changes that can be made (e.g. length, grammar, clarity of argument etc.).
- Seek specific comments on the experimental design and statistical analysis.
- Are there any areas that should be added to the paper but have been overlooked (e.g. recent references)?

HOW DO I ASK OTHERS TO HELP ME?

Ask someone who is likely to offer *constructive* criticism. There is no point giving your work to someone who you know will be unduly negative or positive. Present it to a number of colleagues at a local journal club or research meeting if you can. This will ensure that you hear a range of different views. Difficult questions are particularly useful. They can help identify weaker areas in your study, such as in the way you present your results or argue your case. Take a while to consider carefully the comments that you get, then revise the paper in order to clarify these issues.

HOW DO I GET MY PAPER TO THE JOURNAL?

Send in your paper with the right number of copies and computer disks. Make sure you have included any diagrams and references. Send a covering letter asking the editor to consider your paper for publication. Include in your letter a brief summary of your key findings and state why this might be of interest to the readers of the journal or the editorial team. Normally you are asked by the editor in the *instructions for authors* to state that the paper is not being submitted elsewhere at present. Some journals also ask that you do not present the data in the paper elsewhere (such as poster or oral conference presentations) until the paper is published or rejected by them.

Journals often reply within a few weeks. Some send you an acknowledgement slip on receipt of the manuscript. If you don't hear anything after a few weeks you can telephone or write to find out what progress your paper has made. Even reputable journals can lose submissions or delay returning unsuitable material.

HOW DO I COPE WITH REVIEWS?

Your paper may be accepted subject to changes suggested by the referees. Few journals will publish your work unaltered. Most referees will make sensible suggestions which will improve the quality of the paper. Sometimes you may wish to contest a point and explain your reasoning to the referee through the editor. Once altered, the paper can be returned in its final draft format.

Work is frequently returned with a polite note declining publication. You may be lucky and receive comments from reviewers which help you revise the manuscript for another journal. Sometimes reviews are quite negative. Don't despair! Plenty of authors have felt like this. Some well known leaders in their fields started out by failing to get their ideas accepted (and still do on occasion).

HOW DO I REWRITE THIS PAPER?

If you have ensured that your research has been well-planned to date, someone somewhere will publish your paper if you are determined to keep submitting it and revising it. You may simply need to choose another journal, or you may have to rethink your briefs; choose a different audience or aim for a smaller circulation journal. If, for whatever reason, the research has not been well-planned you may need to go back and change some aspects of the basic research. This may require further data collection to fill in the gaps identified by the referees. You could try reducing the scope of the paper to make a shorter, more focused piece of work. Take note of reviews. The best peer reviews (for you) ask for minor changes – a word here, a shift of emphasis there, or some extra commas and italics. The hardest reviews strongly disagree with your underlying conclusions or question the whole basis of your methodology. Take some advice from your colleagues again. Don't give up at this point after you have come so far. Most papers require alterations after review. Whatever you do, remember to consider your brief, the journal style etc. when it comes to making any changes to your paper.

HOW DO I RESUBMIT THIS PAPER?

The final draft has to be resubmitted according to the editor's instructions. Don't forget to send multiple copies and use the paper's reference number if one has been assigned. When finally accepted, the editor will then send you a proof copy of your paper in exactly the format that it will appear in the journal. You must proof read this within a specified time limit since the journal has a deadline for publication and printing. There is a special shorthand for proof correction marks and some journals will send you this. Normally it is reasonable to make clear changes on the proof copy. The journal will not allow you to do major revisions at this stage. Check names, titles, addresses, spellings, and the detail of data in tables. Remember that your text may have been edited to fit the journal house style. Return your manuscript as soon as possible and certainly within any specified time period.

THE FINAL PRODUCT

Your paper will appear in print within a few months. Some journals will send you offprints, too. If your work interests other researchers they may write to you at your correspondence address asking for a copy. Some commentators may even write to the journal with correspondence referring to your work. In later years you could find your paper cited by other authors. If your target journal is included in computer-based indexes and abstracts, you will find that a reference will also appear there.

At this point you have reached the final satisfying stage of publication. If you have made it this far, you will certainly have the skills and experience to continue publishing your own work. Your publication adds to and modifies the current state of psychiatric knowledge and therefore adds to the research cycle (see Chapter 1).

KEY POINTS

Plan your strategy:

- Which journal is most appropriate?
- Do they publish the type of research I have done?
- Find out about their submissions process.
- Consider discussing the article with the editor.
- Write a clear and structured article of the right length in the journal style.

▶

Consider writing the article with a colleague:

- Complement each others' skills.
- Reduce the workload.
- Set achievable tasks and encourage progress together.
- Seek constructive feedback from others.

If it is rejected:

- Don't give up! What are the other options?
- Seek advice from someone skilled in publication.
- Consider other publishing forums (e.g. as a poster presentation at a Royal College meeting).

Useful telephone numbers and e-mail addresses:

- *Psychiatric Bulletin* and *British Journal of Psychiatry* Tel 0171 2352351 and ask for the Journals Office.
- *British Medical Journal* Tel 0171 3874499. E-mail www.bmj.com

REFERENCES

1. Lewis, S. The right stuff? A prospective controlled trial of trainees' research. *Psychiatric Bulletin*, 1991; **15**, 478–80.
2. Katona, C. L. E., Roberston, M. M. Who makes it in psychiatry: CV predictors of success in training grades. *Psychiatric Bulletin*, 1993; **127**, 27–9.
3. Smith, R. The electronic future: something for everyone. *British Medical Journal*, 1997; **315**, 1696.

Chapter Twelve

Ethical issues in research

Ann Prothero

INTRODUCTION

Research Ethics Committees (RECs) have been in existence since the 1960s. In 1967, The Royal College of Physicians recommended that all research involving patients and normal subjects should undergo ethical review. This proposal was endorsed by the then Ministry of Health and the RECs were set up with the role of reviewing the ethics of all research proposals involving human subjects. Subsequently, further guidelines have been produced by the various medical colleges, medical and nursing professional organizations, international and regulatory agencies and the Department of Health.

Despite the existence of guidance, it is not possible to provide an exact answer to every ethical question raised by research and RECs have the role of providing a view on specific aspects of individual research projects, in the light of local knowledge. Their role could be said to include:

- To protect research subjects from unethical risks, invasions of privacy, inconvenience or expense.
- To facilitate ethically acceptable and scientifically worthwhile research which may for example lead to new and better treatments from which everyone may potentially benefit.
- To protect researchers and the institutions in which research is conducted from allegations of misconduct.
- To enhance public confidence that necessary medical research is being conducted properly.

WHY SUBMIT RESEARCH TO AN ETHICS COMMITTEE?

There is no legislation relating expressly to RECs, nor is there any obligation in law for research to be submitted to them for review. However, there are a number of reasons for submitting research to local RECs (LRECs) for ethical review:

- Department of Health guidance requires NHS bodies to look to an LREC for advice on research to take place in its premises and on its patients.
- Most hospitals and research centres make it an administrative requirement.
- Evidence of ethical approval is required by many professional journals for research which they publish.
- Regulatory authorities require it when assessing data from drugs trials to decide whether to grant market authorization for a product.

PRESENT SYSTEM OF LOCAL RESEARCH ETHICS COMMITTEES

The present system of LRECs was set up in accordance with the Department of Health guidelines contained in circular HSG(91)5. The Committees were established with the purpose of reviewing the ethics of proposed research projects involving human subjects and which takes places broadly within the NHS.

The LREC advises the NHS body under the auspices of which the research is to be conducted. The Department of Health guidance states it is the NHS body itself which is responsible for deciding whether or not the research should take place after taking into account the advice of the Committee. However, no NHS body should agree to a research proposal without the approval of the LREC and no research should be undertaken without the agreement of the NHS body. This guidance applies equally to the researcher already working within the NHS and having clinical responsibility for the patients concerned as to those researchers who have no association with the NHS and its patients beyond the particular research project.

The LREC can advise any NHS body, for example:

- Health Authorities
- Special Health Authorities and
- NHS Trusts.

LRECs can also, by agreement, advise on research which does not involve NHS patients, records or premises and may be undertaken by, for example:

- Private sector companies
- The Medical Research Council or
- Universities.

ESTABLISHMENT

District health authorities (DHAs) were made responsible for the establishment and administrative support of LRECs, even though the

Committee's function is to provide independent advice to any NHS body within the geographical area. LRECs were set up by the District Health authorities (DHAs) after consultation with all the NHS bodies likely to seek advice from them. However, the LREC itself is independent and not representative or beholden to any of the NHS bodies which collaborated in its establishment.

There is usually one LREC in each Health Authority boundary but there may be two in some districts where there is a high workload, possibly originating from two district research centres in its locality. If this is the case, the DHA should have sought the agreement of all the relevant NHS bodies about the respective responsibility of each LREC and ensure that there are administrative arrangements in place so that they work together effectively.

TYPES OF RESEARCH WHICH NEED TO BE SUBMITTED TO AN LREC

Department of Health guidance states that 'The LREC must be consulted about any research proposal involving:

- NHS patients (i.e. subjects recruited by virtue of their past or present treatment by the NHS) including those treated under contracts with private sector companies.
- Fetal material and *in vitro* fertilization involving NHS patients.
- The recently dead, in NHS premises.
- Access to the records of past or present NHS patients.
- Use of, or potential access to, NHS premises or facilities.'

MEMBERSHIP

An LREC should have between 8 and 12 members. It needs a broad range of experience and expertise so that the scientific and medical aspects of research proposals can be reconciled with the welfare of research subjects and broader ethical implications.

Members should be drawn from both sexes and a wide range of age groups. They should include:

- Hospital medical staff.
- Nursing staff.
- General practitioners.
- Two or more lay people.

LREC members are not representative of those groups from which they are drawn. They are appointed in their own right as individuals of sound judgement and relevant experience.

Members who are health professionals should include those involved in active clinical care as well as those experienced in clinical investigation and research. They should be appointed after consultation with the relevant NHS bodies, professional advisory committees and health professional associations. Lay members should be appointed after consultation with the Community Health Council (CHC). At least one lay member should not be associated professionally with health care and should be neither an employee nor an adviser of any NHS body.

Specialist advice can be sought or members can be co-opted onto the committee if there is a professional, scientific or ethical aspect of a research project which is beyond the expertise of the existing members.

The Chairman and Vice-Chairman should be appointed by the health authority from among the members of the Committee after consultation with the relevant NHS bodies. At least one of the posts should be filled by a lay person.

The term of appointment for members should be three to five years and these can be renewed but normally only two terms of office should be served consecutively.

WORKING PROCEDURES

Standing orders covering the frequency of meetings and working procedures should be drawn up. The LREC should always be able to demonstrate that it has acted reasonably in reaching a particular decision. If a research proposal is not approved, the reasons for the decision should be given to the researcher. Conducting business by post or telephone is discouraged and the circumstances in which Chairman's action is appropriate should be clearly laid out.

A register of all proposals submitted to the LREC should be kept. This should not normally be available for public consultation but should be open to NHS bodies for management purposes.

Once a research project has been approved by the LREC the researcher should:

- Notify the Committee, in advance, of any significant proposed deviation from the original protocol.
- Notify the Committee of an unusual or unexpected result which raises questions about the safety of the research.
- Report on the success or difficulty of recruiting subjects.

LREC meetings will normally be private and the minutes taken confidential to the Committee to allow free discussion of the proposals and because members are not representative of any organization.

The LREC should provide an annual report to the DHA and copies should be sent to all NHS bodies which the Committee advises and to the CHC. The annual report should be made available for public inspection.

ISSUES CONSIDERED DURING THE REVIEW PROCESS

The LREC needs a great deal of information to reach a decision on whether the research proposal is acceptable on ethical grounds. The issues raised by a particular research project depend on the nature of the study.

The Department of Health guidance states that the minimum information the Committee will need to know is:

- Has the scientific merit of the study been properly assessed?
- How will the health of the research subjects be affected?
- Are there possible hazards and, if so, adequate facilities to deal with them?
- What degree of discomfort or distress is foreseen?
- Is the investigator adequately supervised and is the supervisor responsible for the project adequately qualified and experienced?
- What monetary or other inducements are being offered to the NHS body, doctors, researchers, subjects or anyone else involved?
- Are there proper procedures for obtaining consent from subjects or where necessary from their parents or guardians?
- Has an appropriate information sheet for the subjects been prepared.

The Committee may ask for additional information such as:

- The type of research – therapeutic or non-therapeutic.
- The intended group of subjects, for example, children, mentally ill.
- Recruitment methods to be used.
- Subject selection criteria.
- Confidentiality or personal health information.
- Compensation arrangements for injury to subjects.
- The regulatory status of any trial drug or device.

LRECs usually have a standard submission form which asks for the information needed by the Committee to come to a decision and usually needs to be accompanied by a protocol, written patient information and consent document.

TYPES OF RESEARCH

All research projects involving human subjects should be submitted to an LREC, including questionnaire studies. However, the LREC, in its standing orders, may specify that certain research, for example, that involving no risk or having a minimal impact on the patient, may be dealt with by the Chairman's action. Research may be divided into two categories:

- Therapeutic, which may be of direct benefit to the individual participant.
- Non-therapeutic, which is unlikely to be of direct benefit to the individual patient although it may advance scientific knowledge. This category may involve research on healthy volunteers as well as patients.

RECRUITMENT OF SUBJECTS

Participation in research must be voluntary and researchers must take care to avoid exerting undue influence over those they invite to take part. *This is particularly important when recruiting subjects in a dependent relationship with the researcher, for example, employees, students, junior hospital staff.*

The researcher must ensure that the subject is aware that:

- Participation is entirely voluntary.
- Deciding not to take part will not affect the future medical care of the patient.
- If they agree to take part they are free to withdraw at any time without needing to give a reason.
- If the research is non-therapeutic, that it will be of no direct benefit to themselves.

Researchers have a responsibility to ensure that, on recruitment and during the study, subjects do not have or acquire a condition which is contraindicated for the study. Participants in non-therapeutic research do not need to be perfectly healthy so long as taking part does not affect their existing condition. Researchers should also be aware of the health status and current medication of all recruits. Agreement should be sought from subjects to approach their own general practitioner about their participation in the study and refusal for this communication should lead to their rejection as a recruit.

INFORMATION FOR PARTICIPANTS

An *information sheet,* to be kept by the subject, should be prepared in the majority of cases to supplement a verbal explanation of the study. It should be written in clear, non-technical language a lay person can understand and avoid the use of jargon. Such an information sheet should include:

- An invitation to take part in the study which makes it clear that it is research.

- An invitation to ask questions or ask for further information.
- Details of the sponsor, supervisor, researcher and how they can be contacted if there are any queries or problems.
- A statement to the effect that participation is *entirely voluntary*, that declining to take part will not affect future care or the patient's relationship with their doctor and that the subject can withdraw at any time without needing to give a reason. Subjects should be made aware that they will be given time to consider their decision. If sudden withdrawal from the study is not advised, this should be clearly explained.
- An explanation of who will have access to personal information and why and the safeguards in place for ensuring confidentiality.
- An honest explanation of the aims of the study, why it is being done and its duration.
- A clear explanation of the methods to be used (e.g. crossover, randomization, double blind and the use of placebo).
- The likelihood of direct benefit to the subject or others.
- An assessment of the potential risks or side-effects, their nature, probability and consequences either physical or psychological.
- The likelihood of discomfort, distress or inconvenience occurring as a result of taking part in the study.
- An explanation of procedures to be used, samples and measurements to be taken and their frequency. It should be clear which of these is not part of routine clinical practice and are required purely for research purposes.
- The nature of alternative treatments (if any).
- What is required of the subject (e.g. abstention from alcohol or driving, withdrawal of other medication, completion of questionnaires, diaries or interviews, cooperation and the provision of personal and medical information).
- The need to contact the subject's GP.
- A contact name and number for assistance or advice.
- Details of any payments or travel expenses.
- The fact that ethical review has taken place without implying that the research is recommended.
- A procedure for compensation or treatment in the case of injury.

CONSENT

Consent should be sought from subjects to participate in research projects. It should be:

- Voluntary.
- Informed.
- From persons able to give consent.

Consent to participate should not be influenced by anxiety that future medical care or the relationship with the researcher, who may be the doctor who is treating the patient, will be adversely affected. Payment to subjects or any other perceived benefit should not be so significant as to be likely to affect willingness to give consent. Subjects should be reassured that they are free to withdraw from the study without giving a reason and without affecting their treatment.

Potential participants should be given sufficient information to allow a decision to be based on an appreciation and understanding of what the study aims to do and what it involves.

Subjects must be able to make a decision on participation based on an understanding of the nature and purpose of the study. Some research subjects may not be able to give consent or communicate a decision because of their physical or mental condition, for example, people who are unconscious, mentally ill, very elderly or have a learning disability (see the section on special groups later in this chapter).

Written consent should be obtained for all but the most minor procedures and certainly for non-therapeutic research. In some cases witnessed consent may be acceptable, for example, people who have intellectual impairment or have language difficulties because of cultural differences but who are, nevertheless, capable of giving consent.

Subjects should be given sufficient time to study the information and reach a decision, possibly after consultation with relatives or their GP. A consent form specific to the research proposal should be signed. This should state that an information sheet has been given, studied and discussed with the researcher and that the subject agrees to participate in the study.

CONFIDENTIALITY

The Department of Health guidelines state, 'that researchers should be asked to confirm that:

- Personal health information will be kept confidential.
- Data will be secured against unauthorized access.
- No individual will be identifiable from published results without their express consent'.

The subject's consent should be sought for the retention of confidential information beyond the end of the study, usually for several years.

EPIDEMIOLOGICAL RESEARCH USING MEDICAL RECORDS

In principle, patients should consent to their medical records being released to research workers. However, sometimes this would be difficult to achieve and an LREC can approve such a study without consent provided that it accepts that the value of the project outweighs the principle that individual consent should be obtained. If a patient has previously stated that he or she would not wish to release their records, then this should be respected.

Such research should be conducted in accordance with current codes of practice of data protection legislation. Consent should also be sought from the health professional responsible for the relevant aspect of the patient's care where possible. After information has been obtained from the medical records, the patient should not be approached without the agreement of the health professional currently responsible for their care.

Certain enquiries and studies, involving only access to patient records, which are in the public interest do not need to be submitted to an LREC for approval. These are:

- The national UK spontaneous adverse reaction reporting scheme (Yellow Card Scheme of the Committee for the Safety of Medicines – CSM).
- Prescription event monitoring (PEM).
- National morbidity surveys.
- Company sponsored post-marketing surveillance studies.

FINANCIAL ASPECTS

Financial aspects of a study which could influence a patient's decision to take part or affect the researcher's judgement in his or her treatment of subjects should be examined by the LREC. These could include not only payments to subjects or researchers but also benefits to an institution or department. However, the resource implications of a research proposal are the responsibility of the management of the NHS body rather than the LREC. Subjects should only be paid for expenses, time and inconvenience reasonably incurred so that there is no inducement to take risks they would not otherwise take or to enrol in too many studies.

COMPENSATION FOR INJURY TO RESEARCH SUBJECTS

Depending on the body sponsoring the research project, varying arrangements can be made for the compensation of subjects injured either negligently or otherwise. Subjects should be aware of the particular arrangements in place before consenting to participation. It is the responsibility of the LREC to ask for evidence that the sponsor has adequate financial backing for compensation arrangements.

The NHS Executive has issued guidance on 'NHS Indemnity – arrangements for clinical negligence claims in the NHS' (HSG(96)48).

This states that:

> 'In the case of negligent harm, health care professionals undertaking clinical trials or studies on volunteers, whether healthy or patients, in the course of their NHS employment are covered by NHS Indemnity. NHS bodies should ensure that they are informed of clinical trials in which their staff are taking part in their NHS employment and that these trials have the required Research Ethics Committee approval.
>
> Apart from liability for defective products, legal liability does not arise where a person is harmed but no-one has acted negligently. An example of this would be unexpected side-effects during clinical trials. In exceptional circumstances (and within the delegated limit of £50 000), NHS bodies may consider whether an *ex gratia* payment could be offered. NHS bodies may not offer advance indemnities or take out commercial insurance for non-negligent harm.'

Private sector companies who sponsor research are usually able to ensure that compensation arrangements are in place for subjects whose health is affected due to participation in a research project. The Association of the British Pharmaceutical Industry (ABPI) has published guidelines for its members on compensation for injury. Details of the provision of compensation should be sought by the LREC.

Participants in research should be made aware of all known risks and the fact that there may be unforeseen risks and the possible difficulties in obtaining compensation.

SAFETY REQUIREMENTS

The Department of Health guidelines state that where a proposal involves the use of drugs, medicines, appliances or medical devices, the LREC should:

- Insist on assurances of the quality and stability of any substance to be administered. This may be done, for example, by requiring details of any relevant clinical trials exemption certificate. It might also be done by requesting a certified statement that any investigations made at the pre-clinical stage have been carried out to the standards required by the Department of Health under the clinical trial exemption scheme.
- Ensure that medical devices at the pre-clinical stage and not covered by the Medicines Act comply with appropriate safety standards and have been manufactured in accordance with Good Manufacturing Practice or under authenticated systems of quality assurance. Where applicable medical devices should conform to the Essential Requirements of the appropriate European Community Directive.
- Require, in submissions involving complex data, a succinct statement and/or an expert summary.

- Seek outside expert opinion if necessary (for example because there was no member of the Ethics Committee who could guide the committee on the particular field to be covered in the study).

DECEPTION

While the deception of participants in research is seen as ethically unacceptable, much psychological research would be made impossible without withholding some of the details about the research hypothesis until after the data have been collected. This is because many psychological processes can be modified by individuals if they are aware that they are being studied. However, the British Psychological Society's guidelines state that, 'the withholding of information or the misleading of participants is unacceptable if they are likely to object or show discomfort or unease after being debriefed. Before conducting such a study, the investigator has a special responsibility to:

- Determine that alternative procedures avoiding concealment or deception are not available.
- Ensure that participants are provided with sufficient information at the earliest stage.
- Consult appropriately upon the way that the withholding of information or deliberate deception will be revealed.

In studies where the participants are aware that they have taken part in an investigation, when the data have been collected, the investigator should provide the necessary information to complete their understanding of the nature of the research.'

RESEARCH ON SPECIAL GROUPS

Children

The College of Paediatrics and Child Health published guidelines on research with children in 1992 based on six principles:

- Research involving children should be supported, encouraged and conducted in an ethical manner.
- Children are not small adults. They have an additional, unique set of interests.
- Research should only be done on children if comparable results on adults could not answer the same question.
- A research procedure which is not intended directly to benefit the child is not necessarily unethical or illegal.

- All proposals involving medical research on children should be submitted to the local REC.
- A legally valid consent should be obtained from the parent or guardian as appropriate. When parental consent is obtained, the agreement of school age children who take part in research should also be requested by researchers.

Young people aged 16 and 17 are legally entitled to consent to treatment and therapeutic research on their own behalf. Children under 16 years of age may also be able to give consent if they have the capacity to understand what is involved. Parental consent should also be obtained in these circumstances. A parent, guardian or another person with legal custody can give consent for a child under 16 to take part in therapeutic research when the child is not competent to do so. However, the refusal of consent by a child competent to make the decision cannot be overridden by a parent or guardian. In the case of non-therapeutic research, parental consent can only be given if the risks to the child are minimal.

Women

The possibility of pregnancy in female research subjects should be considered and the researcher should always justify the recruitment of women of child-bearing age.

Prisoners

The Department of Health guidelines advise that the explicit consent of the Director of Prison Medical Services to the research proposal must always be sought in addition to the consent of the subject.

People with a mental illness or learning disability

While there are problems associated with undertaking research in people with mental illness or learning disability relating to their vulnerability and ability to give consent, these must be balanced against the need to advance the knowledge and treatment in these conditions. The presence of learning disability or mental illness does not necessarily mean that patients are not competent to give free informed consent to research, neither does detention under the Mental Health Act.

However, there will be some patients who are not competent to consent to participation in research (e.g. those with dementia). There is no legal provision for another person (even a relative) to give consent to treatment or medical research on behalf of an 'incompetent' patient. The Royal College of Psychiatrists' guidelines (1990) recommend that:

> 'it would be good practice in most cases for the research worker to discuss the research with one or more close relatives, and discover their views. If there is no relative, or the

patient expresses the wish that his relatives should not be consulted, it may be appropriate to consult an independent person who knows the patient well and will protect his interests (for example, a nurse). The choice of such a person should be approved by the Ethics of Research Committee. These people should attempt to form a judgement, based on the patient's known previous opinions about research and on his recent behaviour, as to whether the patient would be likely to consent were he able to do so. Any patient who indicates refusal either in words or in actions should be excluded from the research whatever opinion is voiced by the others who have been consulted.'

In certain circumstances a court may authorize medical treatment of an incompetent adult, which could include therapeutic research.

KEY POINTS

- Ethical considerations are an important and integral part of the research process involving human subjects.
- The local research ethics committee must be consulted about any research involving NHS patients.
- The local research ethics committee will require a range of information including risks to patients, information given to patients, consent, who the sponsor will be etc.
- If you are in any doubt regarding whether your study needs local research ethics committee approval, contact the Chairman of the committee.

RECOMMENDED READING

1. Bloch, S., Chodoff, P. *Psychiatric Ethics*, 2nd edn. 1991; Oxford Medical Publications, Oxford.
2. Royal College of Physicians of London. *Guidelines on the Practice of Ethics Committees Involved in Medical Research Involving Human Subjects*, 2nd edn. 1990; Cradley Print Limited, Warley.
3. Royal College of Physicians of London. *Research Involving Patients*. 1990; Cradley Print Limited, Warley.
4. Royal College of Physicians of London. *Research on Health Volunteers*. 1990; Cradley Print Limited, Warley.

Chapter Thirteeen

Obtaining research grants

Julie L. Curran

INTRODUCTION

All studies, no matter how small, will have some cost and resource implications. For many studies your time and other resources will be provided 'free' and you will not need to go through the formal process of obtaining funding. However, for many studies finding the funds and resources to conduct research is a perennial problem. In general, one will need to find some dedicated income for any piece of research, since even if you can do the work required in your 'spare' time, money is frequently essential for other staff, paying for investigations, purchasing equipment, statistical advice or even for accessing more efficient computing facilities.

There are a number of key factors that will be common to every successful grant application and these can be summarized as follows:

- Investigate a range of possible sources of funding.
- Make initial contact with funding bodies that may fund research in your area, then get more details from them about what areas of research they are currently funding.
- Write a clear, focused and accurate proposal.
- If rejected, take careful account of any referees' comments before resubmitting.
- There are many possible sources of research funding. However, unless you are applying for a personal fellowship it is probably best to obtain funding from less well known sources rather than immediately applying to the Medical Research Council or Wellcome. Your chances of success are otherwise likely to be small.
- Your chances of success are much higher if you start with small, highly focused grants, and make good use of that money in terms of generating results, and consequently publications (in peer reviewed journals).
- In this manner you establish your own track record, so that when you do graduate to applying to larger, possibly more prestigious sources of

funding, there is something to encourage them to select your proposal over the many other quality proposals received.

Awards are often advertised in major journals such as the *British Medical Journal*. World Wide Web sites and/or postal addresses for several main grant awarding bodies are listed at the end of this chapter. It is also well worth making use of your locally based R&D departments – present in every university and most NHS Trusts. The staff are employed in these departments to help you, and can be especially useful for providing figures for budgets, salary costs and details of local research schemes. Many will also have web sites that you can access remotely – see for example the one provided by the University of Leeds (address at the end of this chapter).

The kind of financial breakdowns provided can be invaluable, since most grant applications will expect you to list:

- Salary costs.
- National Insurance (NI) costs.
- Superannuation costs.
- Institutional overheads.

In general, you will have to adhere to national NHS and University pay scales.

SOURCES OF FUNDING

Personal fellowships

A personal fellowship is usually used to fund an individual, rather than for a specific piece of work. For personal fellowships both the Medical Research Council (MRC) and the Wellcome Trust have well established schemes for providing research training for clinicians.

- These are available to span all stages of career development, so a previous track record in research is not essential.
- Both the MRC and Wellcome provide three-year training grants for clinicians to undertake PhDs as well as the possibility of shorter one year research posts.
- In common with all grant applications, *prompt* submission of the appropriate forms is essential.
- The schemes may have fixed annual or biannual closing dates, or awards may simply be considered at the next committee meeting, but even under these circumstances the committees may only meet four times a year, and there is often a requirement to have applications lodged a minimum period of time before the committee actually meets.
- There are usually certain qualifying conditions that have to be met (e.g. candidates must have qualified within the past ten years, or be

under the age of 35, but if you have sound personal reasons why you feel this condition should be waived in your case, it is always worth a phone call or letter of enquiry to find out if there is any flexbility in the stipulations).

It is also always worth checking if any specific schemes are currently running in your sub-speciality, for instance, the Wellcome Trust currently has a special scheme for research into mental health, and particularly welcomes applications linking basic science to mental health problems. These Fellowships are advertised annually.

Applications frequently require:

- A full curriculum vitae.
- Details of where you intend to do the research.
- Who will supervise you.
- A short note on your intended research.

Selected candidates are often then invited for interview. Other bodies that fund research fellowships include:

- The Lloyds of London Tercentenary Foundation.
- The Royal Society.
- The Lister Institute of Preventative Medicine.
- The Imperial Cancer Research Fund.
- Beit Memorial Fellowships and others.

Competition for most of these is intense, and individuals new to research may, in practice, stand little chance of being successful.

The handbook of the *Association of Medical Research Charities* (published annually) is invaluable in obtaining information about likely sources of funding for project grants (and other forms of grants) and should be considered required reading.

- The 1997/98 edition lists 96 different charities that fund medical research, with budgets ranging from a several thousand pounds to many millions of pounds.
- Some of the charities may have specific requirements that must be fulfilled before they will award you a grant, (a common one is residence in a particular geographical area) but it does mean that if you can fulfil the requirements the chances of success may be quite high.

The other major source of research funding for clinicians is *The NHS Research and Development Scheme*, which is organized on a regional basis.

- The exact form this takes can vary from region to region, but many regions have abolished deadlines for submission of project grants, and will accept them at any time of the year, for consideration at the next committee meeting.

- One general exception to this are the career development fellowships which require you to make an application on your own behalf for the purposes of doing research towards usually either an MD or a PhD.
- As with other major grant awarding bodies the NHS has publicized priorities for funding of research, and these generally fall into line with the targets set out in the government publication 'The Health of the Nation'.
- It is inadvisable to waste time submitting an application which even you can see does not fit into the national priority areas for research funding.

Project grants

A project grant is a grant where the money is provided for a particular piece of research, and not necessarily for any one individual person. If for instance one received a project grant to cover expenses and salary for two years work you could choose to employ whom you wished, unlike a personal fellowship where the person awarded the fellowship must be the individual who does the work and receives the salary. The main bulk of the work in applying for a project grant is the submission of the work you intend to do (usually 4–5 sides of A4). It is essential that you:

- Spend plenty of time writing this section.
- Remove minor errors and spelling mistakes.
- Provide the highest quality research submission you can muster.

When applying for a project grant:

- It should be written bearing in mind the above comments for personal fellowships.
- You must apply to an organization which funds the area of interest.
- You must be keen and sound keen (why should anyone fund your work if you yourself are not passionately committed to, and fascinated by it).
- You are, in essence, selling your ideas to the grant awarding bodies, and they need to be convinced that it will be in their interests to give you the grant.
- Do not promise too much. Not only will it sound unrealistic to experienced reviewers, but it will also stand you in poor stead for future applications if you fail to deliver the goods on this application.

TARGETING YOUR APPLICATION

It is also advisable to discover what the current trends in funding are. Most grant awarding bodies have clearly defined strategies in terms of the research that they would like to see conducted over the next few years, and grant proposals that fall within their priority areas are more likely to be funded. This is not a case of fabricating an interest in an area in order to obtain funding, but more analogous to swimming with the tide rather than trying to battle against it. As an example the MRC's (1996) corporate plan has two major areas of interest to psychiatrists:

- *Mind and Brain* which covers such topics as integration of molecular and cellular biology with physiological and behavioural studies and elucidating the genetic and biological basis of cognitive development and mental health.
- *The Challenge of Ageing* covering areas such as dementias and cognitive decline with age, and improving our knowledge of the health needs of elderly people, and of effective interventions.

In nearly all cases these strategies are publicly available from the grant awarding body concerned. For smaller bodies that may not produce formal published strategies a phone call to the relevant department should elicit such information if it exists.

CONTACTING GRANT AWARDING BODIES

One important principle is make contact with the organization before simply filling in a form and submitting your grant application. Contact may be written, verbal or via e-mail but you must attempt to establish the answers to at least some of the points listed below:

- Is there a corporate plan?
- Are copies of the guidelines for applicants available?
- What percentage of applicants are funded (and less importantly, actual numbers of applicants)?
- Who are the assessors?
- Can I nominate my own referees (assuming the grant is sent for external review), and what form of review process is undertaken?
- How long is it likely to be before a decision is reached?
- What is the submission deadline?

It is always wise to do one's own research into such matters, and not rely on hearsay or rumour, such as 'so and so will only fund you if . . .' followed by a long list of largely anecdotal statements.

HOW A GRANT IS PROCESSED

It is useful to know what will happen to your carefully worded application when it reaches your selected target, as it can be of use when deciding how to plan your strategy for obtaining research funds. Below is listed a common scheme followed more or less by most grant awarding bodies:

- Early informal inquiries are responded to.
- Formal application forms are sent out.
- Returned forms are checked to see that they fulfil any specified conditions, then dispatched to panels of reviewers.
- Reviewers' comments, and application forms are returned to committee.
- Final decisions are made.
- Cheque arrives?!

As well as following the highly stylized format above, most applications will be assessed by the following core criteria, which are not necessarily listed in order of importance, in addition to whether they meet specific conditions, or intend to cover specific areas of work.

- Scientific quality.
- Value for money (do not be greedy in your requests for consumables funding).
- Your research experience and expertise in the field in which you intend to carry out the work.
- Value to users (i.e. mainly to the grant awardees, but also to a wider audience).
- Timeliness – are you performing up to the minute work, or trailing three years behind the leaders in your field?
- Comprehensibility – is the application generally well written with a logical train of thought, and work being proposed?

KEY POINTS

- Apply early, at least six months before you intend to start work.
- Target, and focus your application.
- Check closing dates.
- Read the *British Medical Journal* and *The Lancet* for advertisements for special schemes.
- Double check the application for minor errors, spelling and grammar.
- Ask someone else to read your application for clarity and accuracy.
- Write and rewrite the research section until it is as near perfect as you can achieve.

USEFUL READING

1. Any documentation produced by the grant awarding body you are applying to.
2. *The Association of Medical Research Charities Handbook*. AMRC, 29–35 Farringdon Road, London, EC1M 3JB. Tel. 0171 404 6454.
3. *The Grants Register; Complete Guide to Post-Graduate Funding World-Wide*. Macmillan, London.
4. *Directory of Grant-Making Trusts (UK)*. Charities Aid Foundation, Tonbridge.
5. McFadzean, G. *The Guide to Making Research Applications*. 1997; Centre for Research into Human Communication and Learning, Cambridge.

WEB SITES, POSTAL ADDRESSES AND TELEPHONE NUMBERS

Medical Research Council (MRC)
20 Park Crescent,
London W1N 4AL.
Tel : 0171 636 5422
http://www.mrc.ac.uk

All the other *Research Councils* can be reached via similar web site addresses, substituting the *initials* of the research council in question for *mrc* in the above address.

The Wellcome Trust
210 Euston Road,
London NW1 2BE.
Tel : 0171 611 8828
http://www.wellcome.ac.uk

Association of Medical Research Charities
29–35 Farringdon Road,
London EC1M 3JB.
Tel : 0171 404 6454
http://www.amrc.org.uk

The Lister Institute of Preventative Medicine
Brockley Hill, Stanmore,
Middlesex HA7 4JD.
Tel : 0181 954 6297

The Nuffield Foundation
28 Bedford Square,
London WC1B 3EG.
Tel : 0171 631 0566

The Leverhulme Trust
15–19, New Fetter Lane,
London EC4A 1NR.
Tel : 0171 822 6952

The University of Leeds
RDInfo Information Resource
provides:

- Monthly funding opportunities.
- Training dates and venues.
- Links to funding organizations.

http://www.leeds.ac.uk/rdinfo/

Index

Page numbers printed in *italic* refer to tables: a letter n after a page number indicates a footnote

Adverse reaction reporting scheme, 165
Alta Vista (search engine), 55
Alternative hypotheses, 92
Ambivalence, towards research, 14, 15, 19–20
ANOVA, 107
Anti-research social milieu, 14
Anti-virus software, 127, 128–9, 134
Assertiveness, 20
Assessment, 36–7
Association of Medical Research Charities, 30, 176
  handbook, 172
Association of the British Pharmaceutical Industry (ABPI), guidelines on compensation for injury, 166
Audit, 5
Authorship, 46
Average, 86

Beit Memorial Fellowships, personal fellowships, 172
Best evidence (review guide), 54
Bibliographic software/databases, 65–6
BIDS (database host), *56*, 64–5, 123
Biological sciences research information, 55
Books
  catalogues, 57–8
  handsearching, 64
Boredom, 141
British Psychological Society, guidelines on withholding information, 167

Career development fellowships, 173
Case control studies, *35*
Case reports, as basis for research, 17
Categorical (nominal) data, 84, 90
'Cause and effect' approach, 27, 31
CD-ROMs, 64, 134
Central tendency, 86
Children, research studies on, 167–8
CINAHL, *56*
  predefined search strategies, 60

Classification systems, in psychiatry, 7
Clinical practice
  constant evolution of, 3–4
  as subject for research, 17
Clinical significance, 94
Cochrane Collaboration, 51, 66
Cochrane Controlled Trials Register (CCTR), *56*, 63
Cochrane Database of Systematic Reviews, 54
Cochrane Library, 54, 55, *56*
Cochrane Methodology Database, 66
Cohort samples, *35*
Committee for the Safety of Medicines, Yellow Card Scheme, 165
Community Health Councils (CHCs), 160, 160–1
Compensation, for injury to research subjects, 165–6
Computer skills
  lack of, 13–14, 139
  training courses, 19, 140
Computer software
  anti-virus software, 127, 128–9, 134
  data acquisition/input, 122–3
  data manipulation, 120–2
  data presentation, 124–6
  data storage, 123–4
  desktop publishing, 120
  drawing packages, *121*, 125–6
  numerical processing, 121–2
  presentation graphics, *121*, 125
  spelling and grammatical error checks, 120
  spreadsheets, 100, 112, *121*, 121–2
  statistical analysis, 100, 112, 121, 122
  viruses, 126–9
  voice-recognition, 123
  word-processing, 120, 121, 137
  see also Databases; *and individual software packages*
Computer viruses, 126–9
  anti-virus software, 127, 128–9, 134
  protecting data, 128

Trojan viruses, 128
Computers, 117–37
access to, lack of, 13–14
choosing, 118–20
compatibility, 126
components, 117–18
data acquisition, 122–3
data security, 129–32
desktop, 117–18, 126
e-mail, 124–5
glossary of terms, 134–7
hardware, *118*, 119n
human error precautions, 130–2
multimedia, 118, 136
notebook computers, 136
personal computers, 126
personal protection, 132–4
research tasks, 120–6
see also Computer software; Computer viruses
Conference proceedings, databases, 55, 57
Confidence intervals, 94, 96, 100
Confidentiality, 39, 40–1, 47, 164
research files, 81
Consent, to participation in research, 39–40, 47, 163–4, 168–9
children, 168
Consultants, discouragement from, 13
Continuous data, 84
Controlled trials, *see* Randomized controlled trials (RCTs)
Cost-benefit analysis, 20, 145
Costs, 37–9, 47
literature search/review, 53
on-line services, 64, 65
in research protocols, 80–1
Criticism, constructive, 6, 153, 154
Critique mentality, 37
Crossover trials, *34*

Data analysis, 66
Data Protection Act 1984, 40–1
Data transformation, 92
Database of Abstracts of Reviews of Effectiveness, 54
Databases, *121*, 123–4
access through an intermediary, 65
bibliographic, 65–6
CD-ROMs, 64
conference proceedings, 55, 57
dissertations, 56–7
existing reviews, 54–5
flat-file, 123
free-text, 124
on-line services, 64–5
ongoing research, 55
published articles, 55–6
relational, 123–4
search costs, 53
search strategy, 58–64
searching features, 62–4
textwords and subject index terms, 59–62
World Wide Web (WWW), 54, 55, 65, 137
see also individual databases and database packages
Deception, of research subjects, 167
Descriptive statistics, *see* Statistics, descriptive
Desktop computers, 117–18, 126
Desktop publishing programs, 120
DH-Data, 57
Dialog Corporation, 56, 64
Datastar, 57, 64
Dialog, 64
Digital cameras, 134
Digital video, 125
Disks (computer), *118*
archives, 130, 131–2
back-up copies, 130, 131–2
problems with, 130
security, 130–2
Dissemination, 44–7, 48
Dissertation Abstracts Online, 56
Dissertations, databases, 56–7
Distribution (statistical), 85, 91–2
deviations from normal, 88–9
normal (Gaussian), 85, 89–90, 92
P-values tables, *102–4*
and random variations, 90
t distribution table, *102–3*
District Health Authorities (DHAs), and Local Research Ethics Committees, 158–9
Dot-matrix printers, 134–5
Drawing packages, 121, 125–6
object-based, 126
pixel-based, 125
Drugs, Institute for Study of Drug Dependence library, 58

E-mail, 124–5
  discussion lists, 58
EMBASE (Excerpta Medica), 53, *56*, 59
Employment, effect on research, 15, 144
Epidemiological research, 164–5
Ethical issues, 39–42, 47, 157–69
  confidentiality, 39, 40–1, 47, 164
  consent, 39–40, 47, 163–4, 168–9
  exploitation and participation, 39, 41
  key points, 169
  medical or experimental treatment, 41–2
  Nuremberg Code, 39
  principles, 39
  and research protocols, 39
  see also Local Research Ethics Committees
Ethical practice, as subject for research, 17
Ethics Committees, *see* Local Research Ethics Committees
Ethnography, 32, 35
Euphoria, 141
EXCEL (spreadsheet), 100, 112
Excerpta Medica (EMBASE), 53, *56*, 59
Experiments, 31, *34*
Experts, as information sources, 58
Exploitation of participants, 39, 41
Eyestrain, 133

Family and friends, support from, 145
Fellowships, 171–3
Feminism, objections to traditional research, 32–3
Focus groups, *35*
Frequency distribution, 85
Frustration, 141
Funding, 18–19, 28–9, 30, 37
  lack of, 144
  see also Grants

Gaussian (Normal) distribution, 85, 89–90, 92
Goals, achievable, 22–4
Grants, 170–6
  assessment criteria, 175
  contacting awards bodies, 174
  key factors in applications for, 170–1
  key points, 175
  personal fellowships, 171–3
  processing of, 174–5
  project grants, 173
  sources of, 170–3, 176
  targeting of applications, 173–4
  training grants, 171
Grey literature, 30, 47
  databases, 57
Grounded theory, 33

Harvard style of referencing, 151
Histograms, 85
House style, journals, 150–1
Hypotheses
  alternative hypothesis, 92
  null hypothesis, 27, 92
  in research protocols, 76
  v. research questions, 26
  setting up, 94–5
  testing, 91, 106
  see also Research questions

Idealist (bibliographic database), 66
Ideas for research, lack of, 13
Imperial Cancer Research Fund, personal fellowships, 172
Implications of research, fear of, 15
IMRD (introduction, method, results and discussion) structure model, 45
Index to Theses, 57
Inferential statistics, 83, 90
Information resources
  guides to, *54*
  see also Databases; Experts; Literature search
Information sheets/leaflets, for research subjects, 40, 162–3
Injury to research subjects, compensation for, 165–6
Ink-jet printers, 135
Institute for Study of Drug Dependence, library, 58
Inter-rater reliability, 76
Interest areas, as subject for research, 17–18
Interest in research, 4–5, 7, 24
  lack of, *12*, 14
Internet, 124, 135
  access costs, 53
Internet Service Providers (ISPs), 119–20, 124
Interval data, 84, 90

Interviews, *35*
Irrelevance, of research?, 14
ISI Current Contents database, *56*

Jargon, 45
Job demands, 15, 144
Job interviews, 11
Job plans, research built into, 16
Joint undertaking, 5, 24
Journal clubs, 148
Journals, 149
  choice of, for publication, 148–9
  databases of published articles, 55–6
  handsearching, 58
  house style, 150–1
  instructions for authors, 150, 153
  judging of articles submitted to, 36
  peer-reviewed, 149
  references, 151
  specialist, 149
  submission requirements, 46
  submitting work, 153–4
  see also Publication; Research papers

Keyboards (computer), *118*
Knowledge
  lack of, 139–41
  new, resulting from research, 30
Kruskal-Wallis test, 107
Kurtosis, 89

Language
  jargon, 45
  scientific, 45
  translation facilities, 52
Laptop computers, *see* Notebook computers
Laser printers, 135
Learning disabilities, research studies on people with, 168–9
LED printers, 135
Legal liability, 166
Leverhulme Trust, 176
Libraries
  catalogues, 57–8
  costs, 53
  hospital, 6
  Open Access Catalogues (OPACs), 57
  searching via, 65
  specialist topics, 58
Library of Congress, 58
Life changes, impact of, 15
Lister Institute of Preventative Medicine, 176
  personal fellowships, 172
Literature reviews, 67–8
  costs, 53
  date limits, 52
  existing, 54–5
  geographic limits, 52
  key points, 68
  non-journal articles, 52
  phases in, *51*
  purpose of, 50–1
  resource implications, 51, 53
  systematic approach to, 50–1
  time limits, 52
Literature search, 6, 30, 50–69
  books, 57–8
  data analysis, 66
  documenting the search, 67
  experts as source of information, 58
  grey literature, 30, 47, 57
  handsearching, 58, 64
  for ongoing research, 55
  storing results, 65–6
  translation facilities, 52
  see also Databases
Lloyds of London Tercentenary Foundation, personal fellowships, 172
Local Research Ethics Committees (LRECs)
  communication and records, 160–1
  establishment and support of, 158–9
  information for, 161, 169
  membership of, 159–60
  present system, 158
  and project reviews, 36
  reasons for submission of research to, 157–8
  and research protocols, 81
  types of research for submission to, 159, 161–2
Logistics, in research protocols, 80–1
Lycos (search engine), 55

Mailing lists, 58
Mann-Whitney U test (Wilcoxon rank sum test), 109–10, 113–14, *115–16*
Mean, 86
Mean deviation, 87

Measurement, 7
Median, 86
Medical records, research using, 164–5
Medical Research Council (MRC), 30, 176
  major areas in corporate plan, 174
  personal fellowships, 171–2
Medical Subject Heading (MeSH), 59, 60
MEDLINE, 6, 53, 54–5, *56*, 123
  MeSH (Medical Subject Heading), *59*, *60*
  predefined search strategies via PubMED, 60–1
  search features, 60
  search strategies, 59–62
Mental illness, research studies on people with, 168–9
MeSH (Medical Subject Heading), 59, 60
Methodologies, 31–5
  case control studies, *35*
  choosing, 33–5, 47
  cohort samples, *35*
  crossover trials, *34*
  experiments, 31, *34*
  focus groups, *35*
  grounded theory, 33
  interviews, *35*
  naturalistic (qualitative), 27, 32–3, *35*
  observational studies, *35*
  pluralism, 33, 34, 47
  positivist (quantitative), 27, 31–2, 32–3, 33
  quasi-experimental designs, *34*
  randomized controlled trials (RCTs), 32, *34*, *56*, 60–1
  and research protocols, 76–7
  single case experimental designs, *34*
  surveys, *35*
MINITAB (statistical package), 100, 112
Mode, 86
  unimodal and bimodal curves, 89
Modems, 135
Morbidity surveys, 165
Motivation
  blocks to, *139*
  loss of, 141
  to publish, 147–8
  for research, 10–12, 19–20
Multi-agency research, 29
Multi-professional research, 29
Multimedia computers, 118, 136
Muscat (search engine), 55

National Health Service (NHS)
  Centre for Reviews and Dissemination, 51, 54, 60, 66
  guidance on criminal negligence claims, 165–6
  Research and Development Scheme, 172, 173
  and research ethics, 158–9
National Research Register (NRR), 30–1, *55*
Naturalistic (qualitative) methodologies, 27, 32–3, *35*
Negligence, 165–6
Networks (computer), 136
NHS, *see* National Health Service
Nominal (categorical) data, 84, 90
Non-normal data, non-parametric tests, 105
Non-parametric statistics, *see* Statistics, non-parametric
Normal (Gaussian) distribution, 85, 89–90, 92
Notebook computers, 136
Nuffield Foundation, 176
Null hypotheses, 27, 92
Nuremberg Code, 39

Observational studies, *35*
Open Access Catalogues (OPACs), 57
Order statistics, 106
Ordinal data, 84, 86, 90
  non-parametric tests, 105
Overheads, 38–9
OVID (search interface), *56*, 63, 64

P-values, 92–3, 94
  distribution tables, *102–4*
  interpretation of, *93*, *106*
Page printers, 135
Parametric statistics, *see* Statistics, parametric
Parametric tests, 92
Participants, *see* Research subjects
Peer group pressures, 14
  resisting, 20
Peer review, of project, 36
Peers, support from, 145

Personal computers, 126
Personal fellowships, 171–3
  funding bodies, 171–2
Photocopying costs, 53
Physical sciences research information, 55
Positivist (quantitative) methodologies, 27, 31–2, 33
  feminist objections to, 32–3
Posture, sitting, 132–3
Power calculations, 113
Prescription event monitoring (PEM), 165
Presentation graphics, *121*, 125
Printers, 136
  dot-matrix, 134–5
  ink-jet, 135
  laser, 135
  LED, 135
  page printers, 135
Prisoners, research studies on, 168
Probability, *see* *P*-values
Problem solving, 18–19
Process evaluation, 33–4
Procite (bibliographic database), 66
Procrastination, 15
  overcoming, 21–2
Project grants, 173
Project management, 42–4, 47
  action plan, 42–3, 47
  dissemination, 44–7, 48
  milestones, 43–4
  research outcome management, 42, 43–4, 47
Project protocols, *see* Protocols
Project quality review, 35–7, 47
Project steering groups, 28, 42
Project teams, 29, 47
  multi-professional, 29
Protocols, 39, 70–82
  aims, 76
  as basis for other proposals, 70
  benefits, 70
  content, 75–81
  definitions included in, 77
  dissected in action plan, 42–3
  dissemination of results, 45
  ethical issues specified, 39
  and Ethics Committees, 81
  example and comments on, 77–80
  hypotheses, 76
  introduction/background, 75
  investigator/collaborator list, 75
  key features, *74*
  key points, 81
  length, 73
  logistics, resources and costs, 80–1
  methodology of study, 76–7
  problems with idea of writing, *12*
  purpose, 70
  reasons for, 70
  statistics, 80
  title, 75
  writing, 74
Psychiatry
  19th century 'current thoughts', 2
  change and progress, 3, 3–4
  impediments to progress in knowledge, 6–7
Psychological Abstracts, 55, *56*
PsycINFO, 55, *56*, *59*
PsycLIT, 6, 53, 55, *56*
Publication, 6, 7
  audience, 148–9
  the final product, 155
  instructions for authors, 150, 153
  jointly or individually?, 148
  key points, 155–6
  motivation, 147–8
  personal advantages from, 147
  preparing work for submission, 152–3
  reasons for, 147–8
  starting, 148
  submission for, 46–7, 152–3
  where to publish, 149
  see also Journals; Research papers
PubMED, predefined search strategies, 60–1

Qualitative (naturalistic) methodologies, 27, 32–3, *35*
Quality, project quality review, 35–7, 47
Quantitative (positivist) methodologies, 27, 31–2, 33
  feminist objections to, 32–3
Quartiles, 87
Quasi-experimental designs, *34*

Random-access memory (RAM), *118*
Randomized controlled trials (RCTs), 32, *34*, *56*

Cochrane Controlled Trials Register (CCTR), *56*, *63*
database textwords and subject headings, 60–1
Range, 86–7
Ranks, 106
Ratio data, 84, 90
Reactions to other research, 18
Records, *see* Medical records
Reference Manager (bibliographic database), 66
References, in journals, 151
Rejections
of funding application, 37
of publication attempts, 6
Relevance, of research?, 14
Reliability, 32, 76
Repetitive strain injury (RSI), 132
Research
adverse experiences, 142–3
benefits from, 10–12
failure stages, 138, *142*
interest from, 4–5, 7, 24
as a joint undertaking, 5, 24
maintaining momentum, 138–46
negative views about, 20–1, 143
new knowledge resulting from, 30
obstacles to, external factors, 138–9, 144–5
obstacles to, internal factors, 138, 139–44
place and function of, 1–3, 7
practical implementation requirement, 29
project design problems, 144
skills developed from, 11–12
starting, 5–7, 22–4, 24
starting, blocks to, 12–15, 15–22
therapeutic *v.* non-therapeutic, 162
troika model, 23
see also Local Research Ethics Committees; Motivation; Publication
Research and development (R&D)
NHS scheme, 172, 173
in universities and NHS trusts, 171
Research clubs, 23
Research cycle, 3–4, 7
Research Ethics Committees (RECs), 157
legal position, 157
role, 157
see also Local Research Ethics Committees (LRECs)
Research grants, *see* Grants
Research groups, as learning environment, 147
Research institute libraries, 58
Research knowledge
core knowledge and skills, *140*
past and current, evaluation of, 30–1, 47
Research outcome management, 42, 43–4, 47
Research papers
constructive criticism, 6, 153, 154
proof reading, 155
reading and revising, 152–3
resubmitting, 155
reviews and rejections, 6, 154
rewriting, 154
structure of, 152
see also Journals; Publication
Research phobia, 15
Research protocols, *see* Protocols
Research questions, 26–7, 47
defining, 52
Funnel approach, 71–3
v. hypotheses, 26
identifying, 71–3
length of, 27
need for reading and discussion, 73
refining, 52
resources for answering, 53–8
see also Hypotheses
Research skills, *140*
lack of, 13, 18, 139–41
Research subjects
children, 167–8
compensation for injury, 165–6
consent to participation, 39–40, 47, 163–4, 168–9
deception of, 167
exploitation of, 39, 41
financial aspects, 164, 165
information sheets/leaflets for, 40, 162–3
people with learning disabilities, 168–9
people with mental illness, 168–9

prisoners, 168
recruitment of, 162
rights of, 40
voluntary principle, 162, 163
women, 168
Resources, 37–9, 47
lack of, *12*, 13–14, 18–19, 144
in research protocols, 80–1
see also Information resources
Review, of project, 35–7, 47
Reviews, 17
databases, 54–5
Rotational schemes, 9, 14
Royal College of Psychiatrists, 9
Research Training Coordinators, 23–4
Royal Society, personal fellowships, 172

Safety requirements, research studies, 166–7
Scanners, 136
SciSearch, *56*, 65
SIGLE (System for Information on Grey Literature in Europe), 57
Significance, clinical, 94
Significance testing, 91, 113
SilverPlatter (search interface), 56
Single case experimental designs, *34*
Skewed data, 86, 88–9, 90
non-parametric tests, 105
Social sciences research information, 55
Social SciSearch, *56*, 65
Specialist advice costs, 53
Specialist registrars (SpRs), 9
survey of research done by, 10
training schemes, 9
Spread, 86–8
Spreadsheets, 100, 112, *121*, 121–2
Stakeholders, 28–9, 42, 47
conflicts of interest, 28–9
and project review, 35, 47
Standard deviation, 87–8, 90
Statistical tests
on computers, 122
structure, 92–4
Statistics
analysis methods, 107, 113
descriptive, *see* Statistics, descriptive
inferential, 83, 90
non-parametric, *see* Statistics, non-parametric
parametric, *see* Statistics, parametric
Statistics, descriptive, 83–90
average, 86
categorical (nominal) data, 84, 90
central tendency, 86
continuous data, 84
data, types of, 84
data properties, 84
distribution, 85
frequency distribution, 85
Gaussian (Normal) distribution, 85
histograms, 85
interval data, 84, 90
kurtosis, 89
mean, 86
mean deviation, 87
median, 86
mode, 86, 89
nominal (categorical) data, 84, 90
Normal (Gaussian) distribution, 85, 89–90
ordinal data, 84, 86, 90
quartiles, 87
range, 86–7
ratio data, 84, 90
and research protocols, 80
skewed data, 86, 88–9, 90
spread, 86–8
standard deviation, 87–8, 90
sum of squares, 87
variance, 87
Statistics, non-parametric, 92, 105–16
appropriate situations for use of, 105
computer software, 112
hypothesis tests, 106
Mann-Whitney U test, 109–10, 113–14, *115–16*
order statistics, 106
P-values, 106
parametric *v.* non-parametric tests, 105–6
ranks, 106
significance tests, 113
transformation of data, 92
Wilcoxon rank sum test (Mann-Whitney U test), 109–10, 113–14, *115–16*
Wilcoxon signed rank sum test, 107–9, 113
Wilcoxon signed rank test, 111–12, 114, *114–15*

Statistics, parametric, 91–104
  clinical significance, 94
  computer software, 100
  hypotheses, null and alternative, 92
  hypotheses, setting up, 94–5
  hypothesis testing, 91
  interpretation of results, 93
  non-parametric *v.* parametric tests, 105–6
  P-values, 92–3, 94, *102–4*
  parametric tests, 92
  significance testing, 91
  test statistic, 92
  test structure, 92–4
  see also *t*-tests
Structure, IMRD (introduction, method, results and discussion) model, 45
Submission for publication, 46–7, 152–3
Supervision, access to, 144–5
Supervisors
  effective, attributes of, 145
  training, 29
Support
  from colleagues, peers, family and friends, 145
  lack of, *12*, 13, 18
Surveillance studies, post-marketing, 165
Surveys, 35
  of knowledge/attitudes, as basis for research, 17
System for Information on Grey Literature in Europe (SIGLE), 57

t-tests
  one-sample, 95–6, 101
  paired, 98–100, 101
  t distribution table, *102–3*
  two-sample, 96–8, 101
Tape streamers, 132, 136
Terminology, 7
Test–re-test reliability, 76
Test statistic, 92
Theory development, positivist *v.* naturalist, 33
Thesauri, 59, *60*
Theses, Index to Theses, 57
Time
  lack of, 12, 12–13, 16–17, 143, 144
  prioritization of, 16, 143–4, 145
  research time entitlement, 9, 12–13, 15, 16
Trainees
  lack of technology skills, 139
  research suitable for, 21
  views on training, 18, 139–40
Training
  computer usage, 19, 140
  courses, 140–1
  courses in writing and publishing, 148
  in research, 18
  rotational schemes, 9, 14
  specialist registrars (SpRs), 9
  of supervisors, 29
  training days, 18
Training grants, 171
Transformation of data, 92
Troika model of research, 23

Uncertainty, how to begin research, *12*, 13–14, 17–18
Universities
  courses, 9
  overheads, 38–9

Validity, 32, 76
Vancouver style of referencing, 151
Variables, dependent and independent, 32
Variance, 87
Viruses, *see* Computer viruses
Voice-recognition, 123

Wellcome Trust, 176
  personal fellowships, 171–2
Wilcoxon rank sum test (Mann-Whitney U test), 109–10, 113–14, *115–16*
Wilcoxon signed rank sum test, 107–9, 113
Wilcoxon signed rank test, 111–12, 114, *114–15*
WinSPIRS (search interface), 63
Women, research studies on, 168
Word-processors, 120, *121*, 137
World Wide Web (WWW), 54, 55, 65, 137, 171

Yellow Card Scheme, 165